MCQs in G

MCQs in Geriatric Medicine

Rose Anne Kenny

MB MRCPI

Clinical Registrar, Geriatric Unit, Royal
Postgraduate Medical School, Hammersmith
Hospital, London

Churchill Livingstone

EDINBURGH LONDON MELBOURNE AND NEW YORK 1985

CHURCHILL LIVINGSTONE
Medical Division of Longman Group Limited

Distributed in the United States of America by Churchill
Livingstone Inc., 1560 Broadway, New York, N.Y. 10036,
and by associated companies, branches and
representatives throughout the world.

First published 1985

ISBN 0 443 03174 6

British Library Cataloging in Publication Data

Kenny, Rose Anne
    MCQs in geriatric medicine.—(MCQs)
    1. Geriatrics
    I. Title   II. Series
    618.97   RC952

Produced by Longman Group (FE) Limited
Printed in Hong Kong

Preface

It is a happy paradox that, because of modern advances in medical knowledge and practice, there is today a greater range of clinical problems arising in patients of advanced age — some already known to general medicine, others more specific to the geriatric condition.

MCQs in Geriatric Medicine contains over three hundred multiple-choice questions concerning clinical problems encountered in the elderly. Detailed answers are given for each question and all answers are referenced from up-to-date reviews, original articles and textbooks.

This book is a useful guide to students sitting undergraduate and postgraduate examinations and questions are set out in a similar way to the usual format of the examinations. *MCQs in Geriatric Medicine* is also a useful introduction to clinical problems encountered by those working with the elderly whether in hospital or community practice and encompasses all major clinical areas of medicine in the elderly.

To allow for easy access the answers are arranged on the reverse side of each page, and both questions and answers are grouped according to the particular system under review.

London
1985

Rose Anne Kenny

Contents

1. Cardiology   1   64/175
2. Chest disease   21   43/115
3. Dermatology   33   29/50
4. Endocrinology and metabolism   39   98/260
5. Gastroenterology   61   108/260
6. Haematology   93   61/115
7. Immunology and microbiology   107   49/100
8. Neurology   119   133/345
9. Renal disease   155   62/170
10. Rheumatology   175   26/70
11. Therapeutics   183   9/25
    References   187

1. Cardiology

1.1 *Emboli* causing acute lower limb ischaemia arise from the

- A left atrium in atrial fibrillation
- B left ventricle after myocardial infarction
- C prosthetic heart valves
- D infective endocarditis
- E atrial myxomas

1.2 The following is/are true of acute *lower limb ischaemia*

- A emboli tend to lodge where vessels divide
- B common femoral artery emboli are rare
- C popliteal artery emboli are the most common
- D clotting occurs proximal to the site of impaction
- E dissection of the arterial wall is the commonest cause

1.3 The following clinical features are characteristic of an acute *embolus* to the lower limb

- A absence of pain
- B hyperaemia
- C loss of sensation
- D loss of power
- E enhancement of the pulse proximal to the occlusion

1.4 Diabetes mellitus results in lower limb ischaemic lesions by

- A an increased tendency to atherosclerosis
- B small vessel occlusion
- C vessel infiltration with lymphocytes and giant cells
- D peripheral neuropathy
- E a tendency to infection

1.5 Patients with chronic *lower limb ischaemia* should be advised to

- A stop smoking
- B reduce weight
- C reduce exercise considerably
- D regularly tend to self-care of feet and keep toenails cut short
- E reduce glucose intake

(Answers overleaf)

1.1 A **True**   Acute *lower limb ischaemia* may also result from
    B **True**   *aneurysm* (especially popliteal), tumour, septic
    C **True**   foreign body, paradoxical *embolus*, acute thrombosis
    D **True**   in atherosclerotic vessels (particularly in the elderly),
    E **True**   injury, dissection of the arterial wall and rarer causes
                   such as severe vasospastic disease, frost bite and
                   ergot

                                                    Cecil, pp 319–321

1.2 A **True**   most often in the common femoral artery and
                   sometimes at the aortic, popliteal or iliac bifurcations
    B **False**
    C **False**
    D **False**   clotting occurs distal to the site of impaction
    E **False**

                                                    Cecil, pp 319–321

1.3 A **False**   pain is usually the first symptom
    B **False**   pallor initially, later mottling occurs
    C **True**
    D **True**
    E **True**   There is loss of *pulse* distal to the obstruction and the
                   pulse immediately proximal to the occlusion may be
                   enhanced.

1.4 A **True**
    B **True**
    C **False**   this occurs in Buerger's disease (usually in young
                   men)
    D **True**
    E **True**

                                                    Cecil, pp 319–321

1.5 A **True**
    B **True**
    C **False**   patients should be advised to exercise to the limit of
                   comfort. With encouragement, many patients achieve
                   a gratifying improvement in walking distance by
                   exercise
    D **False**   *foot care* is important but this should be done by a
                   chiropodist to avoid even minor injury
    E **False**   *diabetes mellitus* should be treated if present and a
                   low fat diet implemented if hyperlipidaemic.

                                                    Cecil, pp 319–321

1.6   The following is/are predisposing factor(s) to _digitalis intoxication_

    A   hypothyroidism
    B   hypokalaemia
    C   hypocalcaemia
    D   hypomagnesiumaemia
    E   loop diuretic therapy

1.7   The following is/are side-effects of _digitalis intoxication_

    A   Mobitz type II conduction defect
    B   junctional tachycardia
    C   confusion
    D   psychosis
    E   worsening of heart failure

1.8   The following characteristically cause _sinus bradycardia_

    A   jaundice
    B   constrictive pericarditis
    C   congestive cardiac failure
    D   hypothermia
    E   raised intracranial pressure

1.9   _Sick sinus syndrome_ may refer to the following

    A   persistent inappropriate sinus bradycardia
    B   sinus arrest with no appearance of escape rhythm
    C   bradycardia-tachycardia syndrome
    D   sinoatrial block
    E   digitalis induced sinoatrial block

(Answers overleaf)

1.6 A **True**   *hypothyroidism* is a predisposing factor for *digitalis intoxication* partly because glomerular filtration is depressed and, in addition, the altered activity of the sympathetic nervous system may predispose to the development of cardiac arrhythmias

   B **True**   glycosides inhibit the action of the membrane bound enzyme sodium/potassium ATP-ase, and similar effects occur with hypokalaemia.

   C **True**
   D **True**
   E **True**   hypokalaemia is an important contributory factor in digitalis intoxication, being particularly likely to occur in patients receiving either a benzothiadazine or a loop diuretic such as frusemide or bumetanide (which also causes magnesium depletion)

George, British Medical Journal, 1983

1.7 A **False**   almost any disturbance of rhythm and conduction may occur (with the exception of *Mobitz type II atrioventricular block, parasystole,* and *junctional tachycardia*)

   B **False**
   C **True**
   D **True**   *Confusion* and a psychotic state occur particularly in the elderly
   E **True**

George, British Medical Journal, 1983

1.8 A **True**
   B **False**   constrictive pericarditis and congestive cardiac failure cause *sinus tachycardia*
   C **False**
   D **True**
   E **True**

Other causes of *sinus bradycardia* are congenital, physical training, drugs (digitalis, propranolol, morphine, reserpine), transient increases in vagal tone (vomiting), *myxoedema,* and various infections

Cecil, p. 278

1.9 A **True**   the term *sick sinus syndrome* refers to a constellation
   B **True**   of electrocardiographic findings, all of which have in
   C **True**   common dysfunction of the *sinus node*. The term can
   D **True**   be misleading because in most cases, rather than
   E **True**   representing changes in the sinus node *per se*, it is much more likely that a global atrial disease process is present. Nevertheless dysfunction of the sinus node plays a prominent role in the clinical presentation

Cecil, p. 278

1.10   Which of the following account for resistance across the pulmonary bed

   A   the left ventricle
   B   the left atrium
   C   the pulmonary arterioles
   D   the pulmonary venules
   E   the pulmonary capillaries

1.11   The following is/are causes of _atrial fibrillation_

   A   sick sinus syndrome
   B   jaundice
   C   aortic stenosis
   D   chronic constrictive pericarditis
   E   bacterial endocarditis

1.12   The following is/are true of _Torsades de Pointes_

   A   during sinus rhythm the Q-T interval may be prolonged
   B   disopyramide is the treatment of choice
   C   it may be caused by sino-atrial block
   D   phenothiazines may be causative
   E   it is commonly preceded by an early premature ventricular beat

(Answers overleaf)

1.10 A **False**   the pulmonary arterioles account for up to 50 per cent
      B **False**   of the resistance drop across the pulmonary vascular
      C **True**   bed. Together the pulmonary venules and capillaries
      D **True**   account for the remaining drop. The left side of the
      E **True**   heart does not contribute directly to *pulmonary
                       vascular resistance*

                                                          Cecil, p. 212

1.11 A **True**
      B **False**   jaundice is characteristically associated with
                       bradycardia
      C **False**   is associated with *heart block*
      D **True**
      E **True**

It is also associated with *rheumatic heart disease (particularly
mitral valve disease), ischaemic heart disease, thyrotoxicosis* and
hypertension. It may be associated with atrial septal defect,
pericarditis, chronic lung disease, cardiomyopathy, and
congestive cardiac failure. Not uncommonly, it may appear for
the first time in an elderly patient hospitalised with a febrile
illness such as pneumonia.

                                                          Cecil, p. 270

1.12 A **True**
      B **False**   quinidine, disopyramide, procainamide,
                       phenothiazines and tricyclic antidepressants may all
                       cause this arrhythmia. Treatment is generally directed
                       towards the underlying cause. *Isoprenaline* shortens
                       repolarisation and makes recovery of the ventricles
                       more uniform. Overdrive atrial or ventricular *pacing*
                       also stabilizes rhythm. In some cases propranolol may
                       be indicated provided that a slow basic rate has not
                       initially contributed to the dysrhythmia. Left stellate
                       ganglionectomy is also advocated
      C **True**   Slow cardiac rhythms due to high grade atrio-
                       ventricular block, sino-atrial block, hypokalaemia and
                       hypomagnesemia may all cause the arrhythmia.
      D **True**
      E **False**   The initiating extrasystole is usually late
                                            Cecil, pp 274–275
                       Kenny, Postgraduate Medical Journal, 1984

1.13 *Cardioversion* is indicated in the following circumstances
  A long standing atrial fibrillation
  B digitalis induced ventricular fibrillation
  C atrial fibrillation occurring 2 weeks after open heart surgery
  D sick sinus syndrome
  E pericarditis and atrial flutter

1.14 The following are true of *cardioversion* for *atrial fibrillation*
  A quinine sulphate or disopyramide should be started 24 to 36 hours prior to the procedure
  B embolic phenomena occur in 1 to 3 per cent of patients
  C anticoagulation should be administered for 3 to 6 weeks in all cases
  D electrical shock should not be synchronous with the R wave
  E CK-MB levels rise

1.15 The following changes occur in the ageing *aortic valve*
  A increased stiffness of the cusp bases
  B calcification
  C cusp necrosis
  D lipid accumulation
  E commensural fusion

1.16 The following is/are true of the *conducting system* in ageing
  A the number of pacemaker cells is unchanged
  B atrial fibrous tissue increases
  C the number of bundle of His fibres decrease
  D gross fibrotic changes occur in the atrioventricular node
  E first degree heart block frequently occurs

(Answers overleaf)

1.13 A **False** when *atrial fibrillation* has been present for more than 1 year prior to conversion, 90 per cent of patients will revert to atrial fibrillation after cardioversion

   B **False** excess levels of *digitalis* are a contraindication to cardioversion

   C **False** *cardioversion* is contraindicated less than 6 weeks following open heart surgery

   D **False**

   E **False** whereas it is useful for the elective treatment of atrial flutter which is difficult to treat medically, active inflammatory conditions of the heart, such as pericarditis, are a contraindication

Cecil, p. 288

1.14 A **True** 15–20 per cent will revert after the administration of drugs alone

   B **True**

   C **False** Although the role of anticoagulation has remained somewhat controversial, it is generally agreed that *anticoagulation* should be administered for 3–6 weeks if there is a previous history of *emboli*, or if the patient has a prosthetic heart valve or markedly enlarged left atrium, or is in moderate *congestive heart failure*

   D **False** Failure to synchronise shock with the R wave may result in the R-on-T phenomenon, leading to ventricular fibrillation

   E **True**

Cecil, pp 270–272, 2207

1.15 A **True**   there is a decrease in the number of nuclei in the

   B **True**   fibrous stroma of the valve, accumulation of lipid,

   C **False** degeneration of collagen and calcification of the valve

   D **True**   fibrosa. These changes are mostly seen at the sites of

   E **True**   maximum movement of the valve cusps, and show definite and steady increases with age

Brocklehurst, pp 230–231

1.16 A **False** the number of pacemaker cells in the *sino-atrial node* is reduced

   B **True**

   C **True**   there is loss of fibres in the bifurcating main bundle of His, at the junction of the main bundle and its left fascicles, with lesser loss in the distal bundle branches

   D **False** there is little if any alteration in the atrioventricular node

   E **True**

Brocklehurst, pp 243–244

1.17 **The following physiological changes occur in ageing**

    A reduced *cardiac output*

    B increased *stroke volume*

    C prolonged mechanical systole

    D reduced systolic ejection rate

    E reduced *pulmonary vascular resistance*

1.18 **On *chest radiographs* in a significant number of healthy elderly subjects the following is/are true**

    A the cardiothoracic diameter exceeds 50 per cent of total thoracic diameter

    B the average chest diameter is reduced

    C isolated localised bullae are common

    D vessel shadows are less conspicuous

    E a third demonstrate calcified trachea and/or main bronchi

1.19 **The following is/are true**

    A the incidence of *hypertension* rises with age

    B a systolic pressure of 170 should be reduced to 120 in a 79-year-old man

    C there are age induced changes in baroreceptor activity

    D peripheral venous tone increase with ageing

    E reserpine may induce depression in the elderly

(Answers overleaf)

1.17 A **True**
      B **False**   decreased stroke volume
      C **False**   mechanical systole is unchanged
      D **True**   since stroke volume is reduced and
                      mechanical systole is unaltered, the systolic ejection
                      rate must be reduced
      E **False**   *Pulmonary vascular resistance* is increased

In myocardial failure, the higher the filling pressure the lower the
cardiac output, while in normal old people the higher the filling
pressure the higher the cardiac output. Increased stiffness of the
myocardium would seem a reasonable explanation for the latter
finding.

Brocklehurst, p. 232

1.18 A **True**   in 80 per cent of elderly females and 20 per cent of
                      males over 70 the *cardiothoracic ratio* exceeds 50 per
                      cent — a commonly accepted figure for the upper limit
                      of normal size in younger subjects, but on direct
                      measurements of transverse diameter of the heart
                      there is little difference from that of younger subjects
      B **True**   the increase in cardiothoracic ratio is due to
                      contraction of the thoracic cage, and crude
                      assessment of cardiac enlargement on the basis of 50
                      per cent ratio is of no value in the aged.
      C **False**   isolated localised bullae are occasionally seen in
                      subjects without evidence of generalised *emphysema*
      D **False**   vessel shadows are more conspicuous because of the
                      lower density of rib shadows.
      E **True**

Platt p. 300

1.19 A **True**   systolic pressure increases due to increased vessel
                      wall inelasticity
      B **False**   the treatment of *hypertension* must be undertaken
                      more cautiously than in young or middle aged
                      patients and blood pressure should be reduced very
                      gradually and not below 160–170 mmHg
      C **True**
      D **False**   peripheral venous tone decreases
      E **True**   long-term treatment with reserpine or methyl dopa
                      may induce depressive states in the elderly

Platt, p. 459

1.20   The following is/are true of *aortic stenosis* in the elderly

A   the prevalence is 4 per cent
B   the majority are due to rheumatic valve disease
C   the majority are due to rigid calcification of cusps with normal commissures
D   a third of patients have dyspnoea
E   there is reversed splitting of the second heart sound

1.21   The following may cause *aortic incompetence*

A   bacterial endocarditis
B   dissecting aortic aneurysm
C   calcerous disease of the aortic valve
D   rheumatic heart disease
E   incomplete aortic rupture

1.22   The following is/are true of *syphilitic heart disease*

A   a third of cases are over 70 years
B   it is more frequent in elderly females than males
C   a past history of syphilis is usually obtained
D   cardiac symptoms are frequently present
E   aortic incompetence is clinically severe

1.23   *Senile cardiac amyloidosis*

A   is a form of secondary amyloid
B   is found in over 10 per cent of elderly males
C   occurs most commonly in the left ventricle
D   may cause cardiac failure
E   is never associated with amyloid deposits outside the heart

(Answers overleaf)

1.20 A **True**
    B **False**   20 per cent are definitely due to *rheumatic heart disease*. In these circumstances there is generally coexistent mitral valve disease
    C **True**   apart from rheumatic heart disease there are three other varieties — commissural adhesion and fibrous thickening of the valve cusps giving rise to a triangular or buttonhole orifice, calcific deposition on the aortic aspects of the cusps, giving rise to rigid cusps with a triradiate orifice but normal commissures and thirdly calcification of a congenitally bicuspid valve. The second type is commonest
    D **False**   10 per cent have angina, the majority are asymptomatic
    E **True**

Brocklehurst, pp 253–254

1.21 A **True**   *aortic incompetence* is probably the commonest
    B **True**   valvular lesion in old age. The four commonest causes
    C **True**   in the elderly are *rheumatic heart disease*, calcerous
    D **True**   disease of the aortic valve, syphilitic heart disease and
    E **True**   isolated non-syphilitic aortic incompetence

Brocklehurst, pp 254–255

1.22 A **True**   syphilitic heart disease is rare at any age but 33 per cent of cases are over 70 in recent reports
    B **False**   it is more frequent in old men
    C **False**   a past history of syphilis or antisyphilitic treatment is rarely obtained
    D **True**
    E **True**

Brocklehurst, p. 255

1.23 A **False**   *amyloidosis* of the heart is a separate condition which increases with age
    B **True**   incidences vary between studies but it occurs in at least 12 per cent of men over 80 years and in some studies in up to 60 per cent of females in the 9th decade
    C **False**   it is most frequently found in the left atrial endocardium
    D **True**   if it involves the atria and ventricles
    E **False**   the more extensive cardiac amyloid may be associated with extracardiac deposits but not in sufficient quantity for diagnostic purposes

Brocklehurst, p. 258

1.24 Pressure symptoms due to *aortic dilatation* in the elderly characteristically give rise to

A elevation of the jugular venous pressure
B superior vena cava syndrome
C hoarseness
D dysphagia
E stridor

1.25 The following is/are true of the cardiovascular system in old age

A aortic elasticity increases
B changes in the *aorta* are most apparent in the interna
C *myocardial brown atrophy* is common
D *senile cardiac amyloidosis* occurs in over 70 per cent of subjects
E there is a reduction of pacemaker cells in the *sinoatrial node*

1.26 The following is/are true of *Cheyne-Stokes* respiration

A it occurs in severe heart failure
B it occurs rarely in elderly subjects
C arterial PCO2 reaches its peak during apnoea
D alveolar PO2 reaches its peak during hyperpnoea
E circulation time between the lungs and respiratory centre is prolonged

(Answers overleaf)

1.24 A **True**   pressure on the left innominate vein produces the not
                      infrequent phenomenon of unilateral elevation of the
                      jugular venous pressure
      B **False**
      C **True**   pressure on the left recurrent laryngeal nerve
      D **True**   pressure on the oesophagus just above the
                      diaphragm
      E **False**

                                                      Brocklehurst, p. 230

1.25 A **False**   the elasticity of the human *aorta* declines with
                      decreasing age
      B **False**   changes generally occur in the media — local atrophy,
                      increase in collagen, discontinuity of elastic lamillae
                      and functional changes of elastic tissue
      C **True**   the classical age related change in the myocardia is
                      '*brown atrophy*', a decrease in heart weight
                      accompanied by accumulation of lipofuscin in the
                      myocardial fibres. There is no good evidence that
                      lipofuscin deposition is of any functional importance
      D **False**   12 per cent over 80 years
      E **True**

                                                   Brocklehurst, pp 230–232

1.26 A **True**   some patients in severe *heart failure* display *periodic
                      breathing* characterised by alternate periods of
                      apnoea and hyperventilation
      B **False**   the neurological and cerebrovascular changes of old
                      age predispose to Cheyne-Stokes breathing
      C **False**   cyclic changes in arterial blood gas tensions
                      accompany the waxing and waning respiratory
                      pattern characteristic of Cheyne-Stokes breathing:
                      during apnoea arterial PO_2 reaches its peak whereas
                      arterial PCO_2 reaches its nadir. At the same time
                      alveolar gas tensions are the exact opposite: a low
                      alveolar PO_2 and peak alveolar PCO_2 tension
      D **True**
      E **True**   this slowing of circulation exposes the central
                      respiratory control mechanisms to arterial blood that
                      differs in gaseous composition from that in
                      pulmonary venous blood

                                                           Cecil, p. 141

1.27 In severe *right heart failure*

A anorexia rarely occurs
B cyanosis is usually caused by pneumonia
C the liver is usually enlarged
D jaundice is common
E hydrothorax is more common than in isolated left ventricular failure

1.28 The following is/are true of *oliguria* in heart failure

A it is more commonly associated with left than with right ventricular failure
B urinary sodium concentration is high
C urinary specific gravity is high
D proteinuria is common
E renal casts are rarely detected

1.29 In *mitral stenosis*

A the arterial pulse is anacrotic
B the blood pressure is elevated
C the first heart sound is accentuated
D the apex beat is displaced
E an opening snap follows the first heart sound

1.30 *Mitral regurgitation* occurs in the following

A rheumatic heart disease
B bacterial endocarditis
C Marfan's syndrome
D obstructive hypertrophic cardiomyopathy
E calcification of the mitral annulus

1.31 The following is/are true of *aortic stenosis*

A angina pectoris is often the first symptom
B sudden death occurs in 40 per cent
C the earliest symptom of left ventricular dysfunction is orthopnoea
D acquired stenosis is rare in the elderly
E valve surgery carries a high mortality

(Answers overleaf)

1.27 A **False**   weakness is often marked and accompanied
                      by anorexia, weight loss and malnutrition
      B **False**   *cyanosis* is generally due to sluggish blood flow in the
                      skin vessels and subsequent oxygen extraction
      C **True**   and often accompanied by mild abdominal discomfort
                      and tenderness
      D **False**   *jaundice* is uncommon unless hepatic congestion is
                      associated with long standing *pulmonary congestion*
                      and *pulmonary infarction*
      E **True**

                                                        Cecil, pp 142–143

1.28 A **True**
      B **False**   urinary sodium concentration is low
      C **True**   1.020 to 1.030
      D **True**   but is usually less than 1 g per day
      E **False**   a variety of casts may accompany the proteinuria
                                                        Cecil, p. 144

1.29 A **False**   the arterial pulse is small
      B **False**   blood pressure is low or normal
      C **True**
      D **False**   the heart is not enlarged unless accompanied by
                      mitral regurgitation
      E **False**   the mitral opening snap follows the second heart
                      sound and is audible at the lower left sternal border
                      and apex

                                                        Cecil, p. 195

1.30 A **True**
      B **True**   resulting in rupture of one or more chordae tendineae
      C **True**   again due to rupture of *chordae* tendineae
      D **True**
      E **True**   acquired, heavy calcification of the mitral annulus
                      typically occurs in elderly women and is sometimes
                      associated with significant mitral regurgitation
                                                        Cecil, p. 198

1.31 A **True**
      B **False**   in post-mortem studies of patients who have died
                      from aortic stenosis, death was sudden in about 15
                      per cent. The majority have significant symptoms.
                      Only 3 to 4 per cent die without symptoms
      C **True**   caused by elevated left atrial mean pressure
      D **False**   stenosis resulting from heavy deposition of calcium
                      within the valve leaflets is a common cause of *aortic
                      stenosis* in the elderly. The prevalence of aortic
                      stenosis in geriatric hospital patients is 4 per cent
      E **False**

                                                Cecil, pp 202–203;
                                            Brocklehurst, pp 253–254

1.32 The murmur of *tricuspid regurgitation*

A   occurs early in the course of mitral valve disease
B   results in a decreased jugular V wave
C   is accompanied by a thrill in the lower right sternal border
D   is augmented during expiration
E   is reduced by the Müller manoeuvre

1.33 *Pulmonary emboli* in the elderly

A   are found in 30 per cent of routine autopsies
B   most commonly arise from pelvic veins
C   in hemiplegia arise from the paralysed leg
D   electrocardiographically show S1, Q3, T3, Q AVF pattern
E   are accompanied by calf pain and tenderness

1.34 After *myocardial infarction*

A   coronary artery bypass surgery improves survival in patients with triple vessel disease
B   40 per cent of patients have left main stem disease
C   patients with stenosis of the left anterior descending artery should be considered for angioplasty
D   recurrent angina is a contra indication to coronary angiography
E   reciprocal ST segment depression heralds reinfarction in 25 per cent of cases

(Answers overleaf)

1.32 A **False**   functional *tricuspid regurgitation* occurs late in the
course of *mitral stenosis*
   B **False**   as the right ventricular and mean right atrial pressures
rise in the presence of tricuspid regurgitation, the V
wave increase
   C **False**   there is a thrill over the lower left sternal border and
lower sternum
   D **False**   it is augmented during inspiration
   E **False**   it is augmented during the *Müller manoeuvre* —
attempted inspiration against a closed glottis
Cecil, pp 209–210

1.33 A **True**
   B **False**   in almost all cases *emboli* arise from thrombi in leg
veins, though pelvic veins may be a source in the
obese and after abdominal operations
   C **True**   and may be responsible for non-specific deterioration
in a hemiplegic patient
   D **False**   S1, Q3, T3 pattern without Q AVF
   E **False**   calf pain and tenderness are uncommon in the elderly,
more attention should be paid to oedema, increased
warmth and dilation of superficial veins
Brocklehurst, pp 935–936

1.34 A **True**   *coronary artery bypass surgery* improves survival in
high risk patients, particularly those who have critical
narrowing of the left main coronary artery or triple
vessel disease
   B **False**   up to 10 per cent of patients after infarction have left
main stem disease, and 30 per cent have three vessel
disease
   C **True**
   D **False**   complex *ventricular arrhythmias*, continuing
ischaemia and poor left ventricular function all
indicate high risk patients. Patients with recurrent
angina or evidence of inducible ischaemia should
undergo prompt *coronary angiography* and those
with left mainstem or triple vessel disease and good
left ventricular function should be considered for
bypass surgery
   E **True**   reciprocal ST segment depression in leads remote
from the infarct and developing within 48 hours of the
onset is associated with a 63 per cent incidence of
positive exercise tests and a high likelihood of severe
stenosis in the coronary artery supplying the
reciprocal territory in addition to the disease in the
coronary artery that was responsible for the infarct
Oakley, British Medical Journal, 1983

1.35 *Constrictive pericarditis* **is associated with**

    A   hypoalbuminaemia

    B   hypertension

    C   distant heart sounds

    D   an early diastolic sound

    E   Kussmaul's sign

$$\frac{64}{175}$$

(Answers overleaf)

1.35 A **False**   *ascites* of liver origin is associated with
                       hypoalbuminaemia
      B **False**   *Hypotension*
      C **True**
      D **True**
      E **True**   *Kussmaul's sign* — an inspiratory rise in venous
                      pressure is seen in 40 — 50 per cent of cases

Cecil, pp 137, 305–306

2. Chest disease

2.1 The following is/are true in the elderly

A   In seated males the lower lobes are preferentially ventilated

B   Blood flow is predominantly to the lower parts of the lungs in the upright position

C   Reduced diffusing capacity contributes significantly to arterial hypoxia.

D   Lung compliance increases

E   Chest wall rigidity increases

2.2 The following is/are true

A   The alveolar-arterial oxygen difference increases with age

B   The difference in alveolar-arterial oxygen gradient between old and young subjects is largely abolished by deep breathing

C   Arterial carbon dioxide pressure rises with age

D   Pulmonary vascular resistance is significantly increased at rest in the elderly

E   There is intimal thickening of pulmonary vessels in the elderly

2.3 The following is/are true

A   The bronchial tree is lined by ciliated epithelia as far down as the respiratory bronchioles

B   Tobacco smoking impairs mucociliary action

C   IgG is the predominant antibody in the respiratory tract

D   Viral infections inhibit the rate of clearance of staphylococci

E   Alcohol inhibits the rate of clearance of staphylococci

2.4 Bacteriocidal activity of macrophages is impaired by

A   tobacco

B   acute hypoxia

C   starvation

D   corticosteroids

E   renal failure with acidosis

(Answers overleaf)

2.1 A **False**   in young seated subjects the lower lobes are
                     preferentially ventilated. However in elderly males
                     there is a decreased uniformity in the distribution of
                     ventilation. This difference is abolished by deep
                     breathing. This is probably due to a fall in elastic recoil
                     of the lungs with inefficiency in maintaining patent
                     airways.

   B **True**   as in the young.

   C **False**   the decline in diffusing capacity with age is of little
                     clinical significance. Even in pathologial conditions
                     the diffusion component contributes little to any fall in
                     arterial oxygen.

   D **True**   this is attributable to diminished elastic recoil.
                     (Compliance is the change in volume per unit change
                     in pressure.)

   E **True**   the relative immobility of the rib cage increases the
                     importance of diaphragm and abdominal wall
                     muscles in breathing

                                        Brocklehurst, pp 733–734

2.2 A **True**   there is a progressive fall in arterial oxygen pressure
                     due to increased anatomical shunting

   B **True**
   C **False**   arterial CO_2 pressure does not alter with age
   D **False**   pulmonary vascular resistance at rest is unchanged
                     but it does increase with exercise probably due to
                     diminished elasticity of the pulmonary artery and
                     increased hyalinisation and collagen deposits in the
                     walls of small vessels

   E **True**
                                        Brocklehurst, pp 733–734

2.3 A **True**
   B **True**
   C **False**   secretory IgA is the predominant antibody in the
                     respiratory tract. It differs from serum IgA in its
                     sedimentation rate, amino acid complement and
                     antibody activity

   D **True**   it is 6–8 days before inhibition becomes maximal —
                     corresponding closely with the interval observed
                     clinically between influenza infections and
                     subsequent bacterial pneumonia

   E **True**   also suppresses the cough reflex
                                        Brocklehurst pp, 731, 738

2.4 A **True**
   B **True**
   C **True**
   D **True**
   E **True**

                                        Brocklehurst, p. 738

2.5   In the case of the respiratory system and gram negative organisms

  A   there is usually a predisposing factor for infection
  B   the presence of gram negative organisms always indicates significant infection
  C   sputum bacterial counts usually distinguish between colonization and significant infection
  D   superinfection with gram negative organisms in elderly patients has a high fatality rate
  E   there are specific radiological changes with significant infection

2.6   Acute pulmonary embolism

  A   is excluded if thoracocentesis reveals non bloody effusion
  B   is confirmed by demonstrating a perfusion defect on perfusion lung scan
  C   causes hypoxia due to areas of ateleotasis where perfusion is maintained
  D   causes pulmonary infarction in 50 per cent of cases
  E   is unlikely if the patient's temperature exceeds 38°C

2.7   Static lung compliance is reduced in which of the following conditions?

  A   pulmonary oedema
  B   obesity
  C   asthma
  D   kyphoscoliosis
  E   diffuse interstitial fibrosis

(Answers overleaf)

2.5 A **True**   such as recent or concurrent antibiotic therapy, underlying pulmonary disease and general debility
     B **False**   They may be harmless colonists
     C **False**   Bacterial counts do not distinguish between significant infection and colonisation; the decision is based on clinical progress, radiological appearance and other indicators of active infection
     D **True**   74 per cent in one series
     E **False**   No specific changes in sputum appearance or chest ʻradiograph

Brocklehurst, pp 737–738

2.6 A **False**   the fluid is usually clear and amber
     B **False**   it is only confirmed by demonstrating a perfusion defect on pulmonary angiography. Pulmonary infiltration, local airways obstruction with local reflex vasoconstriction, lung cysts and bullae may all produce perfusion defects on lung scan
     C **True**
     D **False**   pulmonary infarct in less than 20 per cent
     E **False**   temperatures greater than 39°C can occur within the first 48 hours

Cecil, pp 389–394

2.7 A **True**
     B **False**
     C **False**   associated with increased lung compliance
     D **False**   kyphoscoliosis is common in elderly patients and reduces thoracic cage compliance as do skeletal muscle spasticity and pectus excavatum
     E **True**   pulmonary compliance is defined as the change in lung volume for a given change in pressure and it is reduced when the lungs are abnormally stiff due to pulmonary venous congestion, and infiltrative or fibrotic lesions. It is increased in emphysema and asthma. Thoracic cage compliance decreases with age and balances the age related increase in lung compliance

Brocklehurst, pp 733–734
Cecil, p. 340

2.8   The following are associated with the development of bronchiectasis

A   achalasia of the oesophagus
B   measles
C   pulmonary tuberculosis
D   congestive heart failure
E   Recurrent pneumonia

2.9   Bronchiectasis

A   rarely occurs in elderly patients
B   is associated with tuberculosis
C   usually presents with haemoptysis
D   is best treated by continuous antibiotic therapy
E   is frequently associated with sinusitis in elderly patients

2.10   The following is/are true

A   Emphysema is characterised by an increase in the size of air spaces distal to the terminal bronchiole.
B   Chronic bronchitis frequently begins in later life.
C   Chronic bronchitis has an equal sex distribution in the elderly
D   Senile emphysema frequently occurs.
E   Chronic bronchitis is characterised by hypertrophy of the mucosal gland layer.

2.11   Comparing old and young patients with chronic obstructive airways disease

A   the older group has a lesser incidence of purulent sputum
B   hypoxia is significantly more frequent in younger subjects
C   hypercapnoea is significantly more frequent in older subjects
D   40 per cent of elderly subjects have radiological signs of bullae
E   The prognosis of chronic obstructive airways disease is better in older patients when actuarial considerations are allowed for

2.12   Hypertrophic osteoarthropathy may be associated with

A   mesothelioma
B   pulmonary neoplasm
C   biliary cirrhosis
D   bacterial endocarditis
E   fibrosing alveolitis

(Answers overleaf)

2.8   A **False**
      B **True**
      C **True**   particularly in the middle lobe syndrome of Broch
      D **False**
      E **True**

2.9   A **False**   an incidence as high as 13% per cent is found in
                       autopsy studies
      B **True**
      C **False**   usually presents with a chronic productive cough
      D **False**   postural drainage is the most important aspect of
                       treatment
      E **False**   in younger patients bronchiectasis may be associated
                       with sinusitis as part of the cilial dysfunction
                       syndrome

                                                    Cecil, pp 386–387

2.10 A **True**
      B **False**   it is unusual for chronic bronchitis to begin in later life.
                       The incidence of new cases falls during middle age
                       while the number of established cases continues to
                       rise throughout the life span
      C **False**   the condition is more common in men at all ages
      D **False**   it was formerly common to apply this term to chest
                       radiographs but the radiological appearance of the
                       lungs is essentially unchanged in old age, and the
                       term is no longer used
      E **True**

                                               Brocklehurst, pp 740–744

2.11 A **True**
      B **True**
      C **False**   hypoxia and hypercapnoea are both significantly
                       more frequent in younger subjects
      D **False**   7 per cent
      E **True**   tests of ventilatory function, lung volume and
                       diffusing capacity show no difference between young
                       and older groups, indicating that the more marked
                       blood gas changes in the young may be due to better
                       compensation for pathological changes by the old
                                               Brocklehurst, pp 740–744

2.12 A **True**
      B **True**
      C **True**
      D **True**
      E **True**

                                                         Burton, p. 41

2.13 **Malignant tumours which characteristically metastasise to lung are**

    A   sarcomas
    B   breast carcinoma
    C   adrenal carcinoma
    D   renal carcinoma
    E   thyroid carcinoma

2.14 **The following are causes of pulmonary oedema**

    A   mitral stenosis
    B   viral pneumoniae
    C   diffuse intravascular coagulation
    D   paraquat poisoning
    E   septicaemia

2.15 **Cessation of smoking**

    A   reduces the volume of sputum produced
    B   lessens the susceptibility to respiratory infection
    C   improves dyspnoea in all cases
    D   prevents further worsening of airway obstruction
    E   is common in the elderly population

2.16 **The non metastatic effects of bronchial carcinoma include which of the following**

    A   back pain, leg weakness, loss of bowel and bladder control
    B   unilateral ptosis and myosis
    C   arthralgia, limitation of movement and tenderness of wrists and ankles
    D   truncal ataxia, poor co-ordination, and frequent falling
    E   numbness and tingling over the soles of both feet

(Answers overleaf)

2.13 A **True**
      B **True**
      C **True**
      D **True**
      E **True**
Also: bronchial carcinoma, seminoma and chorioepithelioma
Cecil, p. 420

2.14 A **True**
      B **True**
      C **True**
      D **True**
      E **True**
Burton, p. 38

2.15 A **True**
      B **True**
      C **False**   in some patients dyspnoea may improve but this is
                      more likely in heavy cigarette smokers who, after
                      smoking a cigarette, have more pronounced
                      bronchoconstriction than light smokers.
      D **False**   there is no real evidence that stopping smoking
                      prevents further worsening of airway obstruction
      E **True**   there seems to be a spontaneous reduction in tobacco
                      consumption with advancing age, and a concomitant
                      increase in the proportion of ex-smokers in the elderly
                      population
Brocklehurst, p. 743

2.16 A **False**   this is spinal cord compression
      B **False**   this is Horner's syndrome. Both are due to mass
                     effects and not non metastatic manifestations
      C **True**
      D **True**
      E **True**
The non metastatic effects of bronchogenic carcinoma are many
and include hypertrophic pulmonary osteoarthropathy,
spinocerebellar degeneration and peripheral neuropathy. They
also encompass hormonal manifestations of pulmonary
neoplasm
Brocklehurst, p. 749
Cecil, p. 415

2.17 **Pleural fluid glucose concentration of less than 25 mg/dl (<1.5 mmol/l) is compatible with**

    A   pulmonary embolism
    B   tuberculosis
    C   rheumatoid arthritis
    D   pulmonary neoplasm
    E   systemic lupus erythematosis

2.18 **Hypercapnoea may be associated with**

    A   pickwickian syndrome
    B   pneumothorax
    C   barbiturates
    D   chronic bronchitis
    E   hyperventilation

2.19 **Asbestos exposure is associated with an increased incidence of the following**

    A   hilar lymphadenopathy
    B   pleural effusions
    C   mesothelioma
    D   laryngeal carcinoma
    E   gastrointestinal cancer

2.20 **Non-metastatic extra-pulmonary effects of carcinoma of bronchus include**

    A   proximal myopathy
    B   pigmentation
    C   gynaecomastia
    D   hyperglycaemia
    E   red cell aplasia

2.21 **A 69-year-old male who has smoked 20 cigarettes a day for over 50 years presents with haemoptysis of recent onset. Chest radiographs reveal a new right hilar mass. Which of the following serum values might be related to the primary disease.**

    A   sodium 132 mmol/l, potassium 2.9 mmol/l, chloride 94 mmol/l, bicarbonate 34 mmol/l
    B   sodium 118 mmol/l, potassium 3.9 mmol/l, chloride 88 mmol/l, bicarbonate 24 mmol/l
    C   calcium 2.67 mmol/l, phosphate 1.34 mmol/l
    D   thyroxine 14.1 μg/dl, triiodiothyronine uptake 39 per cent
    E   glucose 3.4 mmol/l

(Answers overleaf)

2.17 A **False**   low glucose in pleural fluid is virtually diagnostic of
      B **True**   rheumatoid arthritis if pulmonary neoplasm and
      C **True**   tuberculosis can be excluded
      D **True**
      E **False**

Cecil, pp 356–357

2.18 A **True**   hypoventilation is associated with hypercapnia.
      B **True**
      C **True**
      D **True**
      E **False**

Cecil, p. 494

2.19 A **False**   silica is characteristically associated with hilar
                      lymphadenopathy
      B **True**
      C **True**
      D **True**
      E **True**

Cecil, pp 400–402

2.20 A **True**
      B **True**
      C **True**
      D **True**
      E **True**

Cecil, p. 415

2.21 A **True**   adrenocorticotrophin hormone, antidiuretic hormone
      B **True**   and parathyroid hormone are all secreted by primary
      C **True**   lung neoplasms but neither thyroid stimulating
      D **False**   hormone nor insulin secretion have been reported
      E **False**   with primary lung cancer

Cecil, pp 415–416; 1022–1026

2.22   The following is/are true

A   The incidence of pulmonary tuberculosis has fallen over the past two decades

B   This fall in the incidence of pulmonary tuberculosis is most marked in the older age group

C   Tuberculosis in the elderly is generally due to reinfection

D   There is a decline in tubercular sensitivity with advancing age

E   Pulmonary tuberculosis has a higher mortality in the elderly

2.23   Which of the following findings might be related to an occupational history of working in a shipyard for 10 years, 30 years before presentation?

A   diffuse interstitial fibrosis on chest X-ray

B   encasement of the lung by pleural thickening

C   hilar lymphadenopathy

D   obstruction to airflow, increase in residual volume, reduction in diffusing capacity for carbon monoxide

E   recurrent pleural effusion

43/
/115.

(Answers overleaf)

2.22 A **True**
     B **False**   The fall has been slight in older age groups so that the older people have become an increasingly important part of the total picture
     C **False**   it is due to reactivation of a past-acquired and healed primary tuberculous lesion
     D **True**
     E **True**

Brocklehurst, p. 751

2.23 A **True**
     B **True**
     C **False**
     D **False**   asbestos exposure has not been implicated in causing obstructive lung disease
     E **True**   recurrent pleural effusions are associated with asbestos and do not necessarily indicate an underlying mesothelioma. Asbestos exposure has been causally related to diffuse alveolar fibrosis, bronchogenic carcinoma and mesothelioma, and recurrent pleural effusions

Cecil, pp 440–402

3. Dermatology

3.1 Erythema multiforme is characterised by

A   iris lesions
B   urticaria
C   flaccid blisters
D   crusting lesions
E   fever and malaise

3.2 Erythema multiforme may be precipitated by

A   herpes simplex infection
B   ulcerative colitis
C   mycoplasma infection
D   sulphonamide therapy
E   chlorthiazide therapy

3.3 Seborrhoeic dermatitis

A   occurs more commonly than atopic eczema in the elderly
B   typically involves extensor surfaces
C   is a bullous eruption
D   particularly affects the face
E   is characterised histologically by spongiosis (epidermal oedema)

(Answers overleaf)

3.1 A **True**   these are concentric erythematous rings with pale
                      centres which give a *target* appearance
     B **True**
     C **False**   *erythema multiforme* is characterised by tense
                      blisters. In pemphigus the blisters are flaccid and
                      spread easily with pressure
     D **True**
     E **True**   erythema multiforme often starts dramatically with
                      fever and malaise followed by the appearance of the
                      rash

                                                        Cecil, p. 2290

3.2 A **True**   it may be precipitated by *viral* infections such as
                      herpes simplex or *bacterial* or *fungal* infections
                      including coccidioidomycosis and histoplasmosis;
     B **True**   it may occasionally accompany chronic inflammatory
                      bowel disease or neoplastic disease
     C **True**
     D **True**   drugs are important precipitating factors. The drugs
                      responsible include anti-rheumatic agents such as
                      indomethacin, *phenylbutazone* and *flurbiprofen*,
                      antimicrobial agents such as *sulphonamides* and
                      metronidazole, diuretics such as *chlorthiazide* and
                      psychotropic agents such as *chlorpromazine*
     E **True**

                                                        Cecil, p. 2290

3.3 A **True**   atopic *eczema* becomes progressively less frequent in
                      older age groups
     B **False**   involvement of the flexures is typical, especially the
                      folds around the nose, ears and eyes
     C **False**   the rash is an erythematous eruption, with poorly
                      defined margins and greasy scales
     D **True**   face and trunk
     E **True**   the characteristic feature of the acute phase of all
                      eczematous reactions is the presence of epidermal
                      oedema (spongiosis). This is responsible for the small
                      vesicles that appear. Later, epidermal hypertrophy
                      occurs together with some disturbance of normal
                      keratinisation and causes scaling

                                                     Cecil, pp 2263–2264

3.4   Asteatotic eczema

    A   is intensely itchy
    B   occurs in moist skin
    C   is precipitated by emollients
    D   is most commonly found on the chest and abdomen
    E   is exaggerated by temperature changes

3.5   *Pemphigus* is characterised by

    A   basement membrane antibodies
    B   intraepidermal bullae
    C   a predeliction for involvement of skin on the arms and legs
    D   mucous membrane involvement
    E   circulating immune antibodies

3.6   The following is/are helpful in distinguishing between pemphigoid and pemphigus

    A   oral ulcerations
    B   intraepidermal bullae
    C   an underlying malignancy
    D   serum antibodies localised to the epidermal basement membrane
    E   age of the patient

(Answers overleaf)

3.4 A **True**   the commonest cause of widespread itching in the elderly is dry skin or *asteatotic eczema*. It occurs when ageing skin is lacking in lipid and has increased permeability to water

B **False**   the skin is dry and scaly and may have a 'crazy paving' pattern

C **False**   it is precipitated by any factors tending to increase or decrease transpiration, i.e. washing, detergents, cold weather and centrally heated accommodation. Emollients are recommended as appropriate therapy

D **False**   the shins, back and hands are the commonest sites
E **True**

Brocklehurst, pp 908–909

3.5 A **False**   basement membrane *antibodies* are found in *pemphigoid. Pemphigus* is characterised by immunofluorescent antibodies between epidermal cells

B **True**   the epidermal cells separate, fluid accumulates and flaccid intraepidermal bullae result

C **False**   pemphigus has no specific predilection for site of involvement

D **True**   *mucous membrane* involvement occurs in over 50 per cent of patients and in a third mucous membrane lesions develop before skin lesions

E **True**   antibodies are detected in the skin or in the serum. As with many autoimmune disorders, it is not known whether the antibody is primary or secondary. Remissions and relapses can be forecast by the amount of antibody in the serum

Cecil, pp 2288–2289

3.6 A **True**   oral ulceration is common in *pemphigus* and rare in pemphigoid

B **True**   *pemphigoid* produces subepidermal bullae whereas in pemphigus the *bullae* are in the epidermis

C **False**   the association of malignancy with either pemphigus or pemphigoid is tenuous. Both disorders occur predominantly in the elderly in whom coincidental associations occur frequently

D **True**   serum *antibodies* localised to the basement membrane are found in pemphigoid whereas intercellular epidermal antibody is characteristic of pemphigus

E **False**

Cecil, pp 2288–2289

3.7   Herpes zoster
  A   represents reactivation of a dormant herpes simplex virus
  B   arises from reactivated virus in anterior horn cells
  C   is heralded by pain along one or more dermatomes
  D   is a vesicular eruption
  E   is significantly more common in patients with Hodgkin's
      disease

**3.8   Multinucleated giant cells are seen in scrapings from a blister
      base with Greniser's or Wright's stain in which of the following
      conditions**
  A   herpes simplex
  B   herpes zoster
  C   orf
  D   erythema multiforme
  E   seborrhoeic dermatitis

3.9   _Gereralised pruritus_ is associated with
  A   barbiturate withdrawal
  B   iron deficiency anaemia
  C   megaloblastic anaemia
  D   pemphigoid
  E   lichen planus

3.10   Cutaneous stigmata of arsenic ingestion include
  A   palmar and plantar _keratoses_
  B   melasma
  C   _cafe-au-lait_ spots
  D   rain drop hyperpigmentation
  E   seborrhoeic keratoses

(Answers overleaf)

3.7 A **False**   *herpes zoster* represents reactivation of herpes varicellae virus acquired during a preceding varicella infection, the virus remains alive in the dorsal root ganglion

     B **False**

     C **True**   the first clinical feature is pain and tenderness involving one or more dermatomes, with headache, malaise and fever. After a few days the involved dermatomes are red, oedematous and finally vesiculation and crusting appear

     D **True**

     E **True**   herpes zoster is significantly more common in patients with *Hodgkin's* disease, *leukaemia* and to a lesser extent other malignancies

                                Brocklehurst, pp 42.20–42.21

3.8 A **True**   the *'Tzanch'* smear weights' stain shows
     B **True**   multinucleated giant cells in the vesicles of specific
     C **True**   *viral* infections such as herpes simplex, herpes zoster,
     D **False**   orf, chicken pox, variola and vaccinia
     E **False**
                                Cecil, pp 225–227

3.9 A **True**   in younger age groups, withdrawal symptoms in drug addicts are increasingly important as a cause of generalised *itch*. In the elderly, withdrawal of *barbiturates* or other drugs may provoke a similar but milder reaction

     B **True**

     C **True**   In both *iron deficiency anaemia* and *megaloblastic anaemia*, itch may be a predominant feature but it usually occurs only when the haemoglobin concentration is below 7 g per 100 ml. There are some patients who recognise a recurrence of their anaemia by the reappearance of itching. In *polycythaemia rubra vera*, itch may also be predominant, particularly after a bath

     D **True**

     E **True**

                                Brocklehurst, p. 910

3.10 A **True**
     B **False**   *melasma* is a blotchy pigmentation of the face in women during pregnancy or women taking oral contraceptives

     C **False**   these are characteristically found in *von Recklinghausen's disease* and *tuberous sclerosis*

     D **True**
     E **False**   *Seborrhoeic keratoses* commonly occur in the elderly but are not related to *arsenic* ingestion

                                Cecil, pp 2221–2222

4. Endocrinology and metabolism

4.1 The following changes occur after *standing*

A   a reduction in blood volume of at least 600 ml
B   a fall in haemoglobin
C   a 30 per cent rise in plasma proteins
D   no change in platelet count
E   increased serum iron

4.2 *Alcohol* intake may result in

A   elevated serum lactate levels
B   elevated serum alanine transaminase levels
C   a fall in serum aspartate transaminase levels
D   a fall in serum triglyceride levels
E   a rise in serum gamma glutamyl transpeptidase levels

4.3 In severe illness in the elderly

A   measurements of thyroid function are low because of falls in binding *proteins*
B   a quarter of euthyroid patients have low levels of *thyroid* hormones
C   serum albumin levels are rarely less than 32 g/l
D   dehydration frequently occurs
E   serum globulins are useful predictors of the severity of illness

(Answers overleaf)

4.1 A **True**   ultrafiltration of the blood across the vessel walls occurs in the upright posture so that within half an hour or so a fall of 600–700 ml in the blood volume occurs and results in increases of the order of 10 per cent in large molecules and cells. These changes are seen for all *plasma proteins*, enzymes, haemoglobin, cell counts and platelet count. The effects are generally confined to substances with molecular weights in excess of 5800

    B **False**
    C **True**
    D **False**
    E **True**   changes in other blood substances take place in proportion to the degree of protein binding so that increases are seen for serum iron, calcium, cholesterol, bilirubin, thyroid and other hormones

Hodkinson, p. 9

4.2 A **True**   acutely there are increases in lactate and metabolites of *alcohol*

    B **True**
    C **True**
    D **False**   there may be a marked increase in triglycerides for several weeks after commencing regular intake of alcohol

    E **True**

Hodkinson, p. 11
Mellstrom, Age and Ageing, 1981

4.3 A **True**   marked falls in binding *globulin* and *prealbumin* can occur. Also *triiodothyronine* and *thyroxine hormone* production by the thyroid gland may be markedly reduced

    B **True**
    C **False**   *albumin* falls by only 1 g/1 due to normal ageing; the difference in albumin levels in well old people and ill elderly patients is 7.5 g/l on average

    D **True**
    E **False**   serum globulins are very non-specific markers; *acute phase proteins*—
particularly *C-reactive protein*— are better predictors of severity.

Hodkinson, pp 24–25
Kenny, Age and Ageing, 1984a
Kenny, Age and Ageing, 1985

4.4 In elderly patients

A impaired renal function is usually due to pre-renal causes

B there is a reduction in the ability of the *kidney* to conserve salt and water

C the mean *glomerular filtration rate* rises

D renal concentrating activity is impaired in the presence of urinary infection

E when *renal failure* is mild serum creatinine levels are influenced more by muscle mass than by renal function

4.5 The following is true of the elderly kidney

A the ageing kidney leaks protein

B *proteinuria* is a predictor of mortality

C in urinary tract infections stick testing for proteinuria is a good screening test in the absence of renal impairment

D proteinuria is often associated with congestive cardiac failure

E proteinuria is the rule in glomerulonephritis

4.6 The following is/are true of *serum osmolality*

A the osmotic activity of solutions depends on the number of solute particles

B methods of measurement which use freezing point depressions have coefficients of variance of less than 0.1 per cent

C serum protein normally contributes significantly

D the 95 per cent range of serum osmolality is 269–309 mosmol/kg

E glucose does not contribute to osmolality

4.7 The following is/are true of *hyponatraemia* in the elderly

A the incident of severe hyponatraemia (‹125 mmol/l) is 4.5 per cent of hospital admissions

B symptoms depend on the magnitude not the acuteness of hyponatraemia

C it is commonly caused by intravenous fluids

D when post operative intravenous fluid replacement is necessary, 0.9 per cent saline is preferred to dextrose/saline

E hypertonic saline is never indicated

(Answers overleaf)

4.4   A   **True**   particularly *dehydration* or *congestive heart failure*
      B   **True**   a number of studies have shown that the ability of the
                      elderly kidney to produce concentrated urine is
                      diminished
      C   **False**   the mean *glomerular filtration rate* corrected to
                      surface area of 1.73 m² at the age of 30 is 140 ml/min
                      and this falls to 97 ml/min by 80 years
      D   **True**
      E   **True**

                                                    Hodkinson pp 168–169, 187

4.5   A   **False**   *proteinuria* is always abnormal
      B   **True**   proteinuria is a predictor of mortality in community
                      samples — independent of diabetes mellitus
      C   **True**   but not so when renal failure is present
      D   **True**
      E   **True**

                                                    Hodkinson, p. 189

4.6   A   **True**
      B   **True**   they are very accurate
      C   **False**   because of high molecular weights, proteins have
                      negligible molality despite high concentration and
                      make little direct contribution to *osmolality*
      D   **True**
      E   **False**   serum urea, electrolytes and glucose
                      contribute

                                                    Hodkinson, pp 170–171

4.7   A   **True**

      B   **False**   symptoms of hyponatraemia depend on both the
                      magnitude and the acuteness of electrolyte change
      C   **True**   5 per cent dextrose is one of the commonest causes in
                      hospital in-patients
      D   **True**   in order to maintain the plasma sodium level in the
                      post operative period, 0.9 per cent saline is necessary
      E   **False**   in acute hyponatraemia, the need for treatment is
                      urgent. The plasma sodium should be raised to at
                      least 125 mmol/l within 8 h and this may need to be
                      done by infusion of hypertonic saline. The risk of
                      hyponatraemia in this situation is greater than the risk
                      of circulatory overload.

                                                    Hodkinson, pp 171–173
                                                    Flear, Lancet, 1981

4.8   Severe *hyponatraemia* is characteristically associated with

A   nausea and vomiting
B   confusion
C   convulsions
D   slow relaxation phase of reflexes
E   hemiparesis

4.9   The following is/are true of *thiamine*

A   alcoholism may lead to small intestinal malabsorption
B   urinary assay is the best indicator of chronic deficiency
C   the thiamine pyrophosphate effect is the best laboratory
     measurement of serum activity
D   deficiency occurs in 40 per cent of elderly subject
E   deficiency states should always be treated with multivitamin
     preparations

4.10   *Thiamine* deficiency is characterised by

A   sixth nerve palsy
B   encephalopathy
C   paraplegia
D   cardiac failure
E   nystagmus

4.11   *Vitamin C* deficiency

A   is common in elderly males
B   occurs with vitamin intake of less than 10 mg per day
C   rarely occurs because of poor intake
D   when supplemented, increases urinary hydroxyproline
     excretion
E   is best detected by urine sampling in the elderly

(Answers overleaf)

4.8 A **True**   other physical signs and symptoms in hyponatraemia
     B **True**   are ataxia, focal neurological disorders, general
     C **True**   exhaustion, abdominal cramps, restlessness and
     D **True**   muscle twitching. Thus hyponatraemia may be
     E **True**   misdiagnosed as a *cerebrovascular accident* in an old
                   person

Flear, Lancet, 1981

4.9 A **True**
     B **False**   urinary *thiamine* excretion falls early in deficiency
                   states and therefore cannot distinguish acute from
                   chronic deficiency
     C **True**   *thiamine pyrophosphate* (TPP) is added to the
                   transketolase (TK) assay and the change in activity
                   used to calculate serum thiamine.

$$\frac{\text{TK activity with TPP} - \text{TK activity without TPP}}{\text{TK activity without TPP}} \times 100$$

(greater than 25 per cent implies deficiency states)
     D **False**   reports vary but approximately 6–10 per cent of
                   elderly populations have raised TPP activity. However
                   clinically significant deficiency is rare.
     E **False**   management depends on the underlying cause of the
                   deficiency.

Hodkinson, pp 313–314

4.10 A **True**   brain stem dysfunction results in extraocular *nerve
                   palsies* — particularly 6th nerve
     B **True**
     C **False**
     D **True**
     E **True**   and ataxia

Hodkinson, pp 313–314

4.11 A **True**   in one series 52 per cent of elderly men living at home
                   were deficient
     B **True**   the recommended daily intake is 30 mg
     C **False**   low levels are the result of poor intake — meals on
                   wheels are alarmingly low in vitamin C because of the
                   instability of *ascorbic acid* in meals kept hot for
                   several hours
     D **True**
     E **False**   a number of tests for vitamin C deficiency are
                   available including leucocyte ascorbic acid levels and
                   whole blood levels. Dynamic tests based on urinary
                   output after saturation have not proved practicable in
                   the elderly

Hodkinson, pp 321–322

4.12 *Vitamin C* deficiency is characterised by
    A   delayed wound healing
    B   sheet haemorrhages
    C   periosteal haematoma
    D   microcytic hypochromic anaemia
    E   blue lined gums

4.13 *Folate* deficiency
    A   occurs in high turnover states
    B   is uncommon in the elderly
    C   is associated with affective disorders
    D   is associated with peripheral neuropathy
    E   is often associated with ascorbic acid deficiency

4.14 *Vitamin B12* deficiency is associated with
    A   hypersegmentation of polymorphs
    B   microcytic anaemia
    C   absent ankle tendon reflexes
    D   peripheral neuropathy
    E   confusion

4.15 Elevated *uric acid* levels occur in association with
    A   meals
    B   alcohol
    C   paracetamol
    D   dextran infusion
    E   levodopa

4.16 The following is/are true of *pseudohyponatraemia*
    A   the commonest cause is hyperglycaemia
    B   it may mask true hypernatraemia
    C   plasma osmolality is usually normal
    D   24 hour urinary sodium concentration is usually greater than 40 mmol/l
    E   electrolyte measurement with an ion specific electrode gives a true reading

(Answers overleaf)

4.12 A **True**
      B **True**
      C **True**
      D **False**   characteristically *macrocytic anaemia* but mixed
                     forms occur.
      E **False**   this occurs in lead poisoning; patients with their own
                     teeth develop bleeding gums in severe vitamin C
                     deficiency
                                                    Hodkinson, pp 321–322

4.13 A **True**
      B **False**   deficiency in the elderly has been reported in one-
                     third of hospital admissions, 80 per cent of old
                     people's home residents and 15 per cent of the
                     non-institutionalised elderly in North America
      C **True**
      D **True**   and may be associated with seizure frequency in
                     epileptics and with dementia
      E **True**   both deficiencies frequently coexist in the elderly
                                                    Hodkinson, pp 320–321

4.14 A **True**
      B **False**   *macrocytic anaemia*
      C **True**
      D **True**
      E **True**
                                                    Hodkinson, pp 318–319

4.15 A **True**   a host of other disease states, i.e. *renal failure*,
      B **True**   *myeloproliferative* diseases, and medications may
      C **True**   cause secondary *hyperuricaemia*
      D **True**
      E **True**
                                                    Cecil, pp 1108–1111

4.16 A **False**   hyperglycaemia increases plasma osmolality but the
                     commonest cause of *pseudohyponatraemia* is
                     hyperlipidaemia and hyperproteinaemia
      B **True**
      C **True**
      D **False**   because it is not a true *hyponatraemia* the urinary
                     sodium excretion is normal, i.e. spot sodium
                     concentration is less than 10 mmol/l and 24h sodium
                     excretion less than 20 mmol/l
      E **True**   ultracentrifugation and measurement of sodium in
                     clear plasma or the use of non-specific electrodes give
                     true electrolyte readings
                                                    Flear, Lancet, 1981

4.17   Sick cell syndrome

    A   is secondary to inappropriate ADH secretion
    B   is the commonest cause of hyponatraemia in psychogenic polydipsia
    C   may be accompanied by an osmolality gap of more than 10 mosmol/kg
    D   is associated with weight gain
    E   only occurs in acute illnesses

4.18   Thyroid crisis

    A   frequently accompanies surgery on the thyroid gland
    B   may be mistaken for acute manic psychosis
    C   is associated with hypothermia and tachycardia
    D   may be associated with adrenal insufficiency
    E   is precipitated by fluid overload

4.19   The following are used in the treatment of thyroid crisis

    A   propranolol
    B   propylthiouracil
    C   diuretics
    D   salicylates
    E   hydrocortisone

4.20   Ocular complications of diabetes mellitus include

    A   cataracts
    B   glaucoma
    C   rubeosis iridis
    D   retinal infarction
    E   venous engorgement

(Answers overleaf)

4.17 A **False**   it results from the impaired ability of cellular
                    membranes to constrain organic solutes and the
                    subsequent solute leak into extracellular fluid is
                    accompanied by water molecules. Hyponatraemia
                    results with a solute gap
   B **False**   in *psychogenic polydipsia* hyponatraemia results
                    from the dilutional effect
   C **True**   an osmolality gap greater than 10 mosmol/kg
                    suggests significant solute in the plasma
   D **False**   no weight change
   E **False**   *'Sick cell syndrome'* may occur in association with
                    long-term illnesses

                                                    Flear, Lancet, 1981

4.18 A **False**   patients known to be *thyrotoxic* are prepared
                    appropriately for surgery. Crisis rarely accompanies
                    thyroid surgery today
   B **True**
   C **False**   *hyperthermia* and tachycardia
   D **True**   if untreated, it leads to exhaustion, hypotension and
                    adrenal insufficiency
   E **False**   is precipitated by trauma, infection, *dehydration*,
                    thyroid surgery

                                                       Cecil, p. 1212

4.19 A **True**
   B **True**
   C **False**   patients are frequently dehydrated and require
                    intravenous fluids
   D **False**   *salicylates* increase free thyroid hormones and
                    oxygen consumption — external cooling and
                    acetoaminophen should be used for hyperpyrexia
   E **True**

                                                      Cecil, p. 1212

4.20 A **True**
   B **True**
   C **True**   this new vessel formation over the iris may cause
                    glaucoma
   D **True**   *'Cotton wool spots'*
   E **True**

                                                 Brocklehurst, p. 727

4.21   *Steroid therapy* in elderly patients is frequently associated with

A   hypertension
B   psychosis
C   easy skin bruising
D   infection
E   pyrexia

4.22   The following is/are true of corticosteroid therapy in the elderly

A   cortisone utilisation is increased with age
B   hypercorticoadrenalism occurs at smaller doses than in younger patients
C   osteoporosis frequently occurs
D   long-term low dose therapy is often necessary for polyarthralgia
E   steroids should always be combined with anti-inflammatory agents when treating temporal arteritis

4.23   Ageing is associated with

A   a fall in *haemoglobin* A_1C
B   a rise in glucose tolerance
C   an upward trend in fasting glucose levels
D   decreased insulin metabolic clearance rate
E   prolonged *insulin* half-life

4.24   Normal ageing is associated with

A   impaired peripheral *glucose* uptake
B   fasting superficial venous plasma glucose level of less than 7.0 mmol/l
C   similar results in the oral glucose tolerance test as in younger non diabetic subjects
D   glucose intolerance
E   raised incidence of type 2 *diabetes mellitus*

4.25   *Hypoglycaemia* may occur in association with

A   Beta cell pancreatic tumours
B   fibrosarcoma
C   gastrectomy
D   carcinoid tumours
E   adrenocortical carcinoma

(Answers overleaf)

4.21 A **False**
B **True**
C **True**   skin changes include thinning, striae, easy bruising and poor wound healing
D **True**   bacterial, viral or fungal. Tuberculosis may also complicate *steroid therapy*.
E **False**

Cecil, p. 87

4.22 A **False**   *cortisone utilisation* in the elderly is decreased
B **True**   because of decreased cortisone utilisation
C **True**
D **False**   though frequently used to treat polyarthralgia, *steroid therapy* is unnecessary and should be avoided in elderly patients
E **False**   steroids alone suffice in the majority of these patients

Cecil, p. 87

4.23 A **False**   a rise from 7 per cent at 25 years to over 9 per cent after 70 years of age
B **False**   decrease in *glucose tolerance*
C **True**   but the difference is not significant between elderly and young subjects
D **False**
E **False**   *insulin* half-life, metabolic clearance rate and insulin-glucagon relationships are unaffected by ageing

Hodkinson, pp 209–210

4.24 A **True**   rates of *peripheral glucose uptake* are maintained only at the expense of higher glucose and *insulin* levels
B **True**   fasting levels greater than 7.8mmol/l are diagnostic of diabetes
C **False**   the upper limits in arterialised, venous or superficial venous plasma in the elderly are less than:
13.3 mmol/l (240 mg/dl) from 30–90 min
12.2 mmol/l (220 mg/dl) at 120 min
11.1 mmol/l (200 mg/dl) at 150 min
10.6 mmol/l (190 mg/dl) at 180 min
D **True**
E **True**

Hodkinson, p. 223

4.25 A **True**   insulinoma
B **True**
C **True**   patients who have undergone gastrectomy, gastrojejunostomy or pyloroplasty may develop *hypoglycaemia* after meals
D **True**
E **True**

Hodkinson, pp 230–233

4.26   *Ostemalacia* **is characterised by**
   A   peripheral neuropathy
   B   cerebellar ataxia
   C   proximal myopathy
   D   hirsutism
   E   bone pain

4.27   *Hypothyroidism* **may be associated with**
   A   absent ankle jerks
   B   cerebellar ataxia
   C   proximal myopathy
   D   optic atrophy
   E   large bowel obstruction

4.28   **The following is/are characteristic of** *hypothyroidism* **in older subjects**
   A   confusion
   B   hallucinations
   C   depression
   D   agitation
   E   deafness

4.29   **The following is/are true of anaemia in** *hypothyroidism*
   A   it is present in one-third of patients
   B   it is closely correlated with the severity of hypothyroidism
   C   iron deficiency is the commonest cause
   D   the commonest finding is macrocytosis
   E   low B12 levels are found in 30 per cent of cases

(Answers overleaf)

4.26 A **False**
      B **False**
      C **True**
      D **False**
      E **True**

Brocklehurst, p. 767

4.27 A **True**   initially the relaxation phase of ankle and other *reflex*
                     jerks is delayed and finally ankle jerks may
                     disappear — this is particularly so in *myxoedema*
                     coma where plantar responses may be extensor
      B **True**   particularly trunkal ataxia
      C **True**   although this more commonly occurs with
                     thyrotoxicosis
      D **False**
      E **True**   constipation commonly occurs. Pseudo-obstruction,
                     though a much less common feature of
                     hypothyroidism, is well recognized. The aetiology is
                     unknown

Kenny, Postgraduate Medical Journal 1984
Bahemuka, British Medical Journal 1975

4.28 A **True**
      B **True**
      C **True**   up to two-thirds of patients admitted to a geriatric unit
                     and found to have *hypothyroidism* present a non-
                     specific picture of impaired mobility, apathy and
                     depression
      D **True**   though apathy and *depression* are more common,
                     agitation and anxiety may occur together with
                     hallucinations
      E **True**   in the majority of patients this is not reversible after
                     treatment with thyroxine

Kenny, Postgraduate Medical Journal, 1984
Bahemuka, British Medical Journal, 1975

4.29 A **True**
      B **False**   there is no close correlation between the severity and
                     duration of *hypothyroidism* and the degree of
                     anaemia
      C **False**   iron deficiency and microcytic anaemia occur in less
                     than 5 per cent
      D **True**
      E **False**   low vitamin B12 levels are found in less than 10 per
                     cent of subjects

Brocklehurst, p. 696

4.30 **Binding of thyroxine and triiodothyronine to *thyroid* binding globulin is reduced by**

A   severe illness
B   oestrogens
C   nephrotic syndrome
D   corticosteroids
E   protein losing enteropathy

4.31 **The following is/are true of *thyroid* function in ageing**

A   subjects living at home show no change in serum thyroxine levels
B   plasma thyroid stimulating hormone levels are elevated in females
C   thyroid hormone levels are significantly lower in nursing home than in community subjects
D   thyroid autoantibodies rise
E   hyperthyroidism is better tolerated than in younger patients

4.32 **The following is/are true of *ectopic* Cushing's syndrome**

A   it occurs in 20 per cent of patients with oat cell carcinoma
B   10 per cent of reported cases have pancreatic neoplasm
C   physical changes are invariably present
D   hypokalaemia is uncommon
E   there is usually suppression with high dose dexamethasone

4.33 **The following is/are true of *cervical carcinoma***

A   blood stained vaginal discharge rarely occurs
B   secondary vaginal infection is frequent
C   pain is an early symptom
D   tumour spread is by direct invasion of blood vessels
E   cervical cancers are resistant to radiotherapy

(Answers overleaf)

4.30 A **True**   severe illness is associated with reduced serum
                     protein levels
      B **False**   increased by oestrogens
      C **True**   through renal protein loss
      D **False**
      E **True**

Hodkinson, p. 157

4.31 A **False**   Levels are only unchanged in healthy elderly subjects
                     living at home and on no medication — this does not
                     constitute the majority of elderly at home
      B **True**   in the absence of overt thyroid disease, the plasma
                     thyroid stimulating hormone in men does not
                     increase but in women there is a progressive rise in
                     plasma thyroid stimulating hormone with age which
                     is entirely related to an increasing prevalence of
                     thyroid antibodies
      C **True**   and in hospital in-patients
      D **True**
      E **False**   older people tolerate *hyperthyroidism* poorly and the
                     total thyroxine at diagnosis is lower than in younger
                     patients

Hodkinson, pp 159–160

4.32 A **False**   3 per cent
      B **True**
      C **False**   usually metabolic changes — hypokalaemia and mild
                     proximal *myopathy*
      D **False**
      E **False**   suppression with high dose dexamethasone usually
                     does not occur in *ectopic ACTH* syndrome but does
                     occur in *Cushing's* disease of pituitary origin

Cecil, pp 1022–1026

4.33 A **False**   blood stained *vaginal discharge* is a common
                     presentation — particularly in older subjects
      B **True**
      C **False**   pain is usually a late symptom
      D **True**   tumour spread is by direct invasion of lymph or blood
                     vessels
      E **False**   the majority are treated by radiotherapy

Brocklehurst, p. 665

4.34   *Endometrial carcinoma* **is associated with**
   A   early coitus
   B   reduced fertility
   C   late menopause
   D   obesity
   E   nulliparity

4.35   *Ovarian theca cell tumours*
   A   present with vaginal bleeding
   B   are radiosensitive
   C   are rarely malignant
   D   present early in the majority of patients
   E   are uncommon in the premenopausal period

4.36   **The following occur in association with** *ascorbic acid* **deficiency**
   A   normocytic anaemia
   B   bone pain
   C   subperiosteal haematoma
   D   macrocytic anaemia
   E   splenomegaly

(Answers overleaf)

4.34 A **False**   there is a significant association between *endometrial carcinoma* and the single state
     B **True**
     C **True**
     D **True**
     E **True**

Brocklehurst, pp 665–666

4.35 A **True**   due to endometrial hyperplasia associated with their oestrogen-producing ability
     B **False**   *ovarian tumours* are generally radiation insensitive excepting granulosa cell tumours
     C **False**
     D **False**   in contrast with *endometrial cancer*, 70 per cent of patients with *ovarian carcinoma* present with advanced disease. Pain, abdominal swelling and *vaginal bleeding* are the most frequent initial symptoms
     E **True**   granulosa cell tumours are more common in the premenopausal period (constituting 40–60 per cent of ovarian tumours); theca cell tumours are more characteristic of the ageing female.

Brocklehurst, p. 667

4.36 A **True**   *anaemia*, both normocytic and macrocytic, is multifactorial in origin — there is evidence of both iron and folate deficiency
     B **True**   malaise, weakness and lassitude, aching in the bones and *joints* and perifollicular haemorrhages are early features
     C **True**   this occurs most frequently in infantile scurvy. Loosening of the periosteal attachment leads to capillary bleeding which may dissect the periosteum free over a large area. *Subperiosteal haemorrhages* are most frequently found at the lower end of the femur, upper end of the humerus, both ends of tibia and the chostochondral junctions of the middle ribs
     D **True**
     E **False**

Hodkinson, pp 321–322
Cecil, pp 1370–1372

4.37 **Persistent *vomiting* may result in**
   A   metabolic acidosis
   B   elevated urinary potassium
   C   secondary hyperaldosteronism
   D   hyperkalaemia
   E   saline resistant alkalaemia

4.38 **In an active 70-year-old widow the corrected serum *calcium* was elevated. Likely causes are**
   A   multiple myeloma
   B   Paget's disease
   C   primary hyperparathyroidism
   D   hypothyroidism
   E   thiazide diuretics

4.39 ***Reverse T3 is***
   A   formed by a loss of the iodine atom from 5' position on thyroxine phenotic ring
   B   metabolically inactive
   C   increased following a single dose of dexamethasone
   D   elevated in thyrotoxicosis
   E   elevated in elderly in-patients

(Answers overleaf)

4.37 A **False**   *metabolic alkalosis*
      B **True**
      C **True**   extracellular volume depletion and secondary
                     hyperaldosteronism result from vomiting and
                     contribute to the elevated urinary potassium levels
      D **False**   *hypokalaemia*
      E **True**   *vomiting* leads to extracellular volume contraction
                     and to hydrogen ion loss from which results a
                     metabolic alkalosis. This alkalosis cannot be corrected
                     until the glomerular filtration rate returns to normal
                     (i.e. until volume deficits are restored) by correction
                     with saline administration. *Alkalaemia* may be 'saline
                     resistant' and require additional potassium chloride
                     administration. However, this occurs more commonly
                     in primary mineralcorticoid excess and potassium
                     depletion

                                          Cecil, pp 483, 492–493

4.38 A **True**
      B **False**   immobilised patients with *Paget's disease*
      C **True**
      D **True**   and hyperthyroidism
      E **True**   other possibilities are *lymphoma, leukaemia, vitamin
                     D* excess, sarcoidosis, *steroid* withdrawal and
                     metastases

                                          Burton, p. 152

4.39 A **False**   loss of iodine atom from 5' position results in 3:5:5'
                     triiodothyronine (T3) whereas loss of iodine atom
                     from the pyrol ring produces reverse T3 (3:3':5' —
                     triiodothyronine)
      B **True**
      C **True**   reverse T3 levels rise after surgical operation, in liver
                     disease, starvation and generally in acute and chronic
                     medical illness
      D **True**   in thyroid disease the levels of reverse T3 follow those
                     of T4 and T3
      E **True**   low T3 levels in the elderly hospital inpatient are
                     associated with high levels of *reverse T3*. This is in
                     contrast to the situation in healthy old people where
                     lower T3 values are not accompanied by elevation of
                     reverse T3

                                          Brocklehurst, pp 689–690

4.40 In post menopausal females

A FSH levels decline
B FSH:LH ratio is greater than 1
C LH production declines
D oestradiol levels rise
E androstenedione levels decline

4.41 The following may be elevated in a confused elderly female admitted to hospital after falling

A alkaline phosphatase
B creatine kinase
C bilirubin
D aspartate transaminase
E gamma glutamyl transferase

4.42 The following is/are true of *fat emboli*

A the true fat embolism syndrome is rare in old age
B it classically occurs with fractured neck of femur
C 50 per cent of cases have a transient snowstorm appearance on chest radiograph
D large doses of intravenous heparin are effective
E a petechial rash occurs on day 4 after trauma

(Answers overleaf)

4.40 A **False**   *FSH* and *LH* production increases at the menopause
                       and levels remain high in elderly females
      B **True**   there is on average a 15-fold rise in FSH and 5-fold rise
                       in LH levels. The comparatively greater increase in
                       FSH production results in an FSH:LH ratio of greater
                       than 1. In hypothalamic-pituitary failure the ratio is
                       reversed
      C **False**
      D **False**   *oestrone* and *oestradiol* levels decline
      E **True**   androstenedione is produced at a reduced rate by the
                       postmenopausal ovary

                                                      Hodkinson, p. 247

4.41 A **True**   elevated levels of *creatine kinase, aspartate*
      B **True**   *transaminase* and *bilirubin* are secondary to soft
      C **True**   tissue injury and *bruising. Alkaline phosphatase* rises
      D **True**   approximately 7 days after bony injury
      E **False**

                                      Campbell, Age and Ageing 1981

4.42 A **True**   it characteristically occurs in young men with tibial
                       fractures
      B **False**
      C **True**
      D **False**   *Heparin* has been tried for its lipid clearing properties
                       but proved to do more harm than good
      E **False**   the peak incidence of the petechial rash is at 24 to
                       48 h after trauma. The distribution of the rash is the
                       best clinical clue to the diagnosis — the root of the
                       neck, axillae, anterior chest wall and the fundi.
                       Unfortunately, the rash is only present in 50 to 60 per
                       cent of cases

                                                      Cecil, p. 395
                                      Gosling, Clinical Orthopaedics 1982

5. Gastroenterology

5.1 The following is/are true of gastrointestinal disease in the elderly

A functional disease rarely occurs in patients over 65
B mortality is a third of that due to cardiovascular disease
C constipation usually indicates colonic neoplasm
D depression may present with abdominal pain
E serious infection may present with little or no fever

5.2 Zenker's diverticulum

A occurs in the lower oesophagus
B is caused by achalasia
C results in aspiration pneumonia
D may present with dysphagia
E results in a neck mass

5.3 The following is/are true of achalasia

A it most commonly first appears in middle age
B there is excessive relaxation of the lower oesophageal sphincter
C the response to cholinergic drugs is exaggerated
D it predisposes to oesophageal carcinoma
E the number of ganglion cells in Aüerbachs plexus is increased

(Answers overleaf)

5.1 A **False**   a considerable proportion of gastrointestinal symptoms in the elderly are functional. In one study of 300 patients over 65 years, 56 per cent had functional disease

    B **True**
    C **False**   constipation is common
    D **True**
    E **True**   physical signs may frequently be atypical. Serious infection may present without fever or leukocytosis and an abdominal mass may be due to *faecal impaction* or a *distended bladder*

Platt, p. 2
Kenny et al, Age and Ageing, 1984a

5.2 A **False**   *Zenker's diverticulum* develops through the fibres of the cricopharyngeus muscle. It generally appears when the patient is elderly

    B **False**   the development of the diverticulum is thought to be due to failure of relaxation of the cricopharyngeal sphincter with premature closure of the sphincter after initial relaxation and before swallowing is complete.

    C **True**   when the diverticulum is large, symptoms include regurgitation, foul breath, gurgling, aspiration and a neck mass

    D **True**   *dysphagia* is localized to the upper oesophagus
    E **True**

Platt, p. 6

5.3 A **True**   there is less bias towards the older age groups in this condition than with carcinoma, but it continues to produce symptoms, especially dysphagia throughout life

    B **False**   the manomeric abnormalities are hypertension and failure of relaxation on swallowing of the lower oesophageal sphincter and absence of co-ordinated peristalsis in the body of the oesophagus

    C **True**
    D **True**   long-standing *achalasia* predisposes to carcinoma, which has been reported in from 2 to 7 per cent of patients, due to chronic stasis and inflammation

    E **False**   ganglion cells in *Aüerbachs plexus* in the body of the oesophagus are diminished in number. Changes in the vagus nerve and in its dorsal motor nucleus in the brain have been described and raise the question of whether disease is primarily in the oesophagus or in the brain and/or vagus nerve

Platt, p. 6
Brocklehurst, p. 511

5.4 **The following is/are causes of abnormal *gut flora***

- A chronic hepatitis
- B Polya partial gastrectomy
- C pernicious anaemia
- D systemic lupus erythematosis
- E autonomic neuropathy

5.5 **The following is/are recognised causes of a hard knobbly *liver***

- A Riedel's lobe
- B syphilis
- C cirrhosis
- D metastases
- E brucellosis

5.6 **The following is/are recognised causes of hepatocellular carcinoma**

- A cirrhosis
- B arsenic
- C nitroamines
- D aflatoxin
- E vinyl chloride

5.7 **The following is/are characteristically associated with *hepatosplenomegaly***

- A tricuspid stenosis
- B myelofibrosis
- C chronic myeloid leukaemia
- D pernicious anaemia
- E hepatic metastases

(Answers overleaf)

5.4 A **False**
    B **True**   this results in a loop system and together
with malfunctioning gastrojejunostomy and
pernicious anaemia, is responsible for *bacterial
overgrowth* secondary to abnormalities of gastric
function

    C **True**
    D **False**   *systemic sclerosis* is characteristically associated with
abnormal bacterial flora due to abnormal gut motility
as are autonomic neuropathy, vagotomy and
ganglion blocking agents. Systemic lupus does not
result in abnormalities in gut motility

    E **True**

Brocklehurst, pp 529–531
Mc Evoy, British Medical Journal 1983

5.5 A **False**
    B **True**
    C **True**   *cirrhosis* with hepatoma
    D **True**
    E **False**
Brucellosis and Reidel's lobe are both associated with
hepatomegaly but not a hard knobbly liver. Other causes are
polycystic liver and hydatid cysts

Cecil, pp 795, 799, 812
Burton p. 53

5.6 A **True**   Vinyl chloride and arsenic both cause angiosarcoma
    B **False**   of the liver. Anabolic androgens are also associated
    C **True**   with hepatocellular carcinoma
    D **True**
    E **False**

Cecil, pp 812–813
Burton p. 59

5.7 A **False**   other causes characteristically associated with
    B **True**   *hepatosplenomegaly* in older patients are Budd-Chiari
    C **True**   syndrome, reticuloses and amyloidosis
    D **True**
    E **False**

Cecil, pp 857–858, 911
Burton, p. 53

5.8 **The following is/are recognised complications of *parenteral nutrition***

A fluid overload
B acidosis
C vessel thrombosis
D fungal infection
E pneumothorax

5.9 **The following characteristically cause *hyperchlorhydria***

A pernicious anaemia
B subtotal gastrectomy
C iron deficiency
D increasing age
E gastric ulcer

5.10 **Serum *gastrin* levels are elevated in**

A Zollinger-Ellison syndrome
B achlorhydria
C folate deficiency
D gastric surgery with bypass enterostomy
E duodenal ulcer

5.11 **A common cause(s)s of calcification on *abdominal radiographs* in elderly patients is/are**

A costal cartilages
B cysticercosis
C phleboliths
D faecoliths
E visceral calcification

5.12 **The following are long-term complications of *gastrectomy***

A stomal ulcer
B iron deficiency anaemia
C myopathy
D constipation
E pulmonary tuberculosis

(Answers overleaf)

5.8 A **True**   fluid overload and electrolyte imbalance frequently
                    complicate *parenteral nutrition* in older patients.
                    There are a host of complications due to excess or lack
                    of nutrients including hypoglycaemia,
                    hyperosmolar syndrome, dehydration, allergic
                    reactions and deficiency states
     B **True**
     C **True**
     D **True**
     E **True**

there are a number of complications of venous catheterisation
including vessel thrombosis, infection (especially yeast or fungal),
pneumothorax, air embolism, vessel perforation and febrile
reactions to pyrogens in the tubing

Cecil, pp 1384–1386

5.9 A **False**   all are associated with hypochlorhydria.
     B **False**   *Hyperchlorhydria* may occur in association with
     C **False**   *peptic ulceration.* Other causes of *hypochlorhydria* are
     D **False**   *gastric carcinoma, gastric polyposis, atrophic*
     E **False**   *gastritis*, pellagra and radiation

Burton, p. 64

5.10 A **True**
     B **True**
     C **False**
     D **True**
     E **True**

Cecil, pp 642
Burton, p. 64

5.11 A **True**
     B **False**   calcification in the abdominal wall by cysticeri is a rare
                     cause of calcification on an abdominal radiograph
     C **True**
     D **True**
     E **True**

5.12 A **True**
     B **True**   *vitamin B12* and *folate* deficiency also occur
     C **True**   secondary to *osteomalacia*
     D **False**   post prandial diarrhoea
     E **True**   recrudescence of pulmonary tuberculosis is
                    associated with a history of previous gastrectomy

Brocklehurst, p. 517

5.13   **The following is/are causes of *acute pancreatitis***

A   hypocalcaemia
B   hyperthermia
C   morphine
D   steroids
E   thiazide diuretics

5.14   **The following is/are associated with steatorrhoea due to *pancreatic insufficiency***

A   osteomalacia
B   keratomalacia
C   hypoalbuminaemia
D   subacute combined degeneration of the cord
E   hypoprothrombinaemia

5.15   **The following is/are true of *pancreatic carcinoma***

A   most arise from the head of the pancreas
B   most carcinomas originate from ductular tissue
C   pancreatic carcinoma is decreasing in incidence
D   Whipple's procedure is a good palliative measure when resection for cure is impossible
E   pancreatic scanning with 75 Selenium is a useful initial screening test

5.16   **The following is/are true of *pancreatic carcinoma***

A   hypoglycaemia frequently occurs
B   it occurs less frequently than benign tumours of the exocrine pancreas
C   it frequently presents with painful progressive jaundice
D   it is often associated with mental symptoms such as depression or anxiety
E   the 5-year survival is 30 per cent

5.17   **The following differentiate *Crohn's disease* from *ulcerative colitis***

A   crypt abscesses
B   skip lesions of normal colonic mucosa
C   rectal sparing on barium enema
D   inflammatory changes in the rectal mucosa
E   perianal abscesses

(Answers overleaf)

5.13 A **False**   *hypercalcaemia* can cause acute *pancreatitis*
     B **False**   *hypothermia*
     C **True**
     D **True**
     E **False**

Cecil, pp 733–737

5.14 A **True**   *vitamin A* deficiency, *vitamin D* deficiency and *vitamin*
     B **True**   *K* deficiency are all associated with malabsorption of
     C **True**   fat soluble vitamins in pancreatic insufficiency.
     D **False**   However, although *vitamin B12* absorption is reduced
     E **True**   by about 50 per cent in patients with *pancreatic
                    insufficiency*, this is insufficient to prevent deficiency
                    syndromes leading to *subacute combined
                    degeneration of the cord*

Cecil, pp 678–703

5.15 A **True**   70 per cent of *pancreatic carcinomas* occur in the head
                    of the pancreas
     B **True**   most carcinomas are adenocarcinomas arising from
                    the ductular cells
     C **False**   the incidence of pancreatic carcinoma has been
                    increasing
     D **False**   there is a high mortality and morbidity associated
                    with *Whipple's procedure* (pancreatic duodenectomy)
                    and it is generally unacceptable as a palliative
                    procedure particularly in older subjects
     E **False**   the test is unreliable

Cecil, pp 739–742

5.16 A **False**   25–50 per cent of patients have *diabetes mellitus*
     B **False**   Benign tumours of the pancreas are rare
     C **False**   the characterisitic presentation is of painless,
                    progressive jaundice
     D **True**
     E **False**   the 5-year survival is 1–2 per cent

Cecil, pp 739–740

5.17 A **False**
     B **True**   only *Crohn's disease* shows skip areas of normal
                    mucosa between segments of involved bowel.
     C **False**   in ulcerative colitis, the rectum may appear normal
                    with barium enema. However, rectal biopsy usually
                    shows inflammatory changes
     D **False**
     E **False**   perianal abscesses, crypt abscesses and mucosal
                    ulcerations may occur in both disorders.

Cecil, pp 699–700

5.18   Which of the following is/are associated with *oesophageal cancer*

A   Plummer-Vinson syndrome
B   achalasia
C   cigarette smoking
D   Barrett's oesophagus
E   previous squamous carcinoma of the head and neck

5.19   *Intestinal ischaemia*

A   only occurs with complete venous or arterial occlusion
B   frequently results in rectal ischaemia
C   is improved by the use of alpha-adrenergic agents
D   commonly involves the small bowel, splenic flexure and descending colon
E   inevitably occurs with occlusion of a main mesenteric vessel

5.20   An elevated breath hydrogen level after oral administration of 50 g of lactose is found in which of the following

A   normal ageing
B   jejunal diverticuli
C   adult coeliac disease
D   pancreatic insufficiency
E   cholestyramine administration

5.21   A 75-year-old female presents with an 8-year history of *rectal bleeding*. On examination she has large prolapsed internal haemorrhoids with overlying superficial ulceration. The most appropriate management for this patient is/are

A   submucosal injection with a sclerosing agent
B   surgical incision and expression of clot
C   rubber band ligation
D   anal dilatation
E   frequent suppositories and stool softeners

(Answers overleaf)

5.18 A **True**
B **True** 2–7 per cent of cases with long standing *achalasia* develop carcinoma
C **True**
D **True** *Barrett's oesophagus* describes columnar epithelium above the gastro-oesophageal junction which may result from oesophageal reflux and predisposes to *oesophageal cancer*
E **True**

Cecil, p. 629
Brocklehurst, p. 513

5.19 A **False** it may occur in non-occlusive ischaemia such as cardiogenic shock, haemorrhage or septicaemia
B **False** the rectum has an extensive collateral blood supply from the iliac arteries and is rarely affected. Occasionally, an area of demarcation may be seen on proctosigmoidoscopy between normally perfused rectum and ischaemic sigmoid colon
C **False** vasoconstrictors such as alpha-adrenergic agents reduce internal blood flow in order to support systemic blood pressure
D **True**
E **False** the occlusion of one main mesenteric vessel does not inevitably result in *intestinal ischaemia*. Generally two of the three main vessels are occluded before ischaemia occurs.

Cecil, pp 720–722

5.20 A **False**
B **True**
C **True** because of carbohydrate malabsorption and subsequent carbohydrate metabolism in the colon
D **False** lactose metabolism is normal in pancreatic insufficiency
E **False** lactose metabolism is normal during cholestyramine therapy
In the *hydrogen breath test*, the undigested disaccharide lactose enters the colon where bacterial fermentation occurs. Hydrogen is produced, absorbed, and then measured in the breath by chromatography

Cecil, pp 685–687
Platt, p. 16

5.21 A **True**
B **False** this would result in severe bleeding
C **True**
D **True**
E **False** disease of this advanced degree is unlikely to respond to such simple measures

Cecil, p. 747

5.22 **The following is/are features of the *superior mesenteric artery syndrome***

    A   weight gain
    B   lower gastrointestinal obstruction
    C   fixed upper gastrointestinal obstruction
    D   aneurysm of the superior mesenteric artery
    E   symptomatic relief in the prone position

5.23 **The following may cause *faecal incontinence***

    A   constipation
    B   ischaemic colitis
    C   oral iron therapy
    D   rectal prolapse
    E   arteriosclerotic dementia

5.24 ***Faecal impaction* is characteristically associated with**

    A   ischaemic colitis
    B   chronic constipation
    C   an empty rectum
    D   faecal incontinence in association with the gastrocolic reflex
    E   semi-formed faeces

(Answers overleaf)

5.22 A **False** weight loss
     B **False** upper gastrointestinal obstruction which is not fixed
                  and varies with changes of position, i.e. hands and
                  knees and prone
     C **False**
     D **False** *superior mesenteric artery obstruction* is a reversible
                  obstruction of the third portion of the duodenum as it
                  passes between the superior mesenteric artery and
                  the fixed retroperitoneal structures. It
                  characteristically occurs with marked weight loss and
                  is partially relieved by positional changes
     E **True**

                                          Cecil, pp 722–723

5.23 A **True**   *constipation* of long-standing leads to *faecal
                  impaction*. The constipating mass becomes gradually
                  dehydrated and hard and the resulting scyballa, by
                  irritating the mucosa of the colon and rectum, cause
                  an outpouring of mucous
     B **True**   any disorder causing diarrhoea in an elderly person
                  may result in faecal incontinence
     C **True**
     D **True**   due to disruption of the anal sphincter
     E **True**   results in neurogenic incontinence
                                          Brocklehurst, pp 541–543

5.24 A **False** *ischaemic colitis* is associated with diarrhoea and
                  faecal incontinence
     B **True**
     C **False** the rectum is however empty in 11 per cent of
                  incontinent patients and 27 per cent of continent
                  patients in long stay geriatric wards
     D **False** with neurogenic incontinence, soiling occurs perhaps
                  once or twice a day in association with the gastrocolic
                  reflex and a formed stool is passed. When *faecal
                  impaction* results in incontinence the patient tends to
                  be continually lying in a mass of semi of unformed
                  faeces
     E **True**

                                          Brocklehurst, p. 542

5.25   The following is/are true of the *temporomandibular joints* in the elderly

A   radiographs of the joint rarely show any lesion
B   there is crepitus on joint movement
C   remodelling of the joint surface is common
D   a high proportion have degenerative joint changes
E   symptoms rarely occur

5.26   The following is/are true of *Sjogren's syndrome*

A   xerostomia is uncommon in the elderly
B   it is usually associated with an autoimmune process
C   parotid gland secretion is seldom affected
D   dysphagia rarely occurs
E   symptoms result from acinae atrophy

5.27   The following are common causes of *dysphagia* in the elderly

A   aneurysm of the aortic arch
B   diffuse oesophageal spasm
C   achalasia
D   pseudobulbar palsy
E   oesophageal stricture

(Answers overleaf)

5.25 A **False** radiographs often show marginal erosions and flattening of the joint surfaces
   B **True**   there may be crepitus or clicking on joint movement, pain in the masticatory muscles, limitation of opening and tenderness of the joint area
   C **True**   the remodelling appears to be more related to functional factors than to age
   D **True**   histological studies on post-mortem material have shown that a high proportion of joints of the elderly have changes of a degenerative nature comparable with those of osteoarthrosis
   E **False** symptoms are very common in the elderly

   Brocklehurst, pp 501–502

5.26 A **False** *xerostomia* and *keratoconjunctivitis sicca* are frequently associated with enlargement of the parotid and/or lacrimal glands.
   B **False** although in younger subjects *Sjogren's* is usually associated with evidence of an *autoimmune disorder*, in the elderly there is no such correlation and the disorder results from acinar atrophy rather than chronic inflammation
   C **False**
   D **False** *dysphagia* is quite common and may be associated with post cricoid narrowing or web formation
   E **True**

   Brocklehurst, pp 502, 509

5.27 A **False** aneurysms of the arch and descending *aorta* are recognised causes of dysphagia and regurgitation but they do not commonly cause dysphagia
   B **True**   symptoms are intermittent and comprise *dysphagia* and retrosternal pain which might resemble cardiac pain
   C **True**   there is less bias towards older age groups in this condition than with carcinoma
   D **True**   the commonest cause of dysphagia is pseudobulbar palsy due to cerebrovascular disease
   E **True**

   Brocklehurst, pp 513

5.28   The following is/are true of *hiatus hernia*

A   it occurs with increasing frequency in later years
B   there is a greater frequency of the condition in females
C   paraoesophageal type is the most common
D   25 per cent are asymptomatic
E   surgical treatment is usually indicated

5.29   Adenocarcinoma of the oesophagus

A   arises in 10 per cent of patients with Barrett's (columnar) epithelium
B   most commonly presents with progressive dysphagia
C   may be associated with persistent chest pain
D   is best treated by radiotherapy
E   is associated with nail bed clubbing

(Answers overleaf)

5.28 A **True**   in one large survey 18 per cent of patients were less than 50 years of age whilst 28 per cent were over 70 years

B **True**

C **False**   the sliding type is commonest; here the oesophagogastric junction moves up through the diaphragmatic hiatus into the chest and produces a bell shaped deformity

D **True**

E **False**   only rarely is surgery contemplated in the elderly. In some patients with severe oesophagitis in whom surgery is not possible, low dose irradiation to the gastric parietal cell area may sufficiently reduce the acid production to allow the inflammation to respond to simple medical measures

Brocklehurst, pp 511–512

5.29 A **True**   adenocarcinoma of the oesophagus arises in 10 to 15 per cent of patients with columnar epithelium and is associated with chronic reflux oesophagitis. Transitional stages of columnar epithelium from atypia to adenoma and carcinoma in situ have been described beside *Barrett's epithelium*

B **True**   over a 6 or 8 month period until only liquids can be taken

C **True**   the *dysphagia* may be accompanied by a steady, boring chest pain which signals mediastinal involvement and inoperability

D **False**   40 per cent of malignant oesophageal tumours cannot be destroyed with conventional 6000 rad therapy. Adenocarcinomas only occasionally respond to radiotherapy and are not as radio-sensitive as squamous cell carcinomas

E **True**   *nail bed clubbing* can be seen with both benign and malignant oesophageal tumours

Cecil, pp 629–630
Brocklehurst, p. 513

5.30 Schatzki's oesophageal ring

A frequently produces symptoms
B is associated with iron deficiency anaemia
C causes dysphagia for solid foods
D is located in the upper third of oesophagus
E is best seen at endoscopy

5.31 The following is/are true of *dysphagia* due to *moniliasis*

A odynophagia is common
B rapid weight loss may occur
C biopsy of an ulcerated area shows invasive hyphae
D cytological washings are normal
E Radiographic changes commonly occur

(Answers overleaf)

5.30 A **False**   it produces symptoms infrequently but in a characteristic manner. Every 3 or 4 months, after a bolus of meat or bread, the patient will complain of dysphagia and total inability to swallow solids or liquids. The bolus will be regurgitated and then the patient can continue to eat normally

   B **False**   an acquired web located at the post cricoid area is associated with iron deficiency anaemia

   C **True**

   D **False**   *Schatzki's ring* is located in the terminal oesophagus, has a symmetrical opening and is usually at the junction between squamous and normal transitional or columnar epithelium

   E **False**   the lower oesophageal ring is not well seen with the rigid endoscope, as the lower portion of the oesophagus cannot be distended enough to force the ring into prominence

                                    Cecil, pp 630–631

5.31 A **True**   infection of the mucosa leads to odynophagia of a rather marked degree. *Dysphagia* for both solids and liquids usually accompanies the odynophagia and can be of such intensity that weight loss is rapid

   B **True**

   C **True**   it may be confused clinically with herpes virus infection which shows characteristic histological nuclear changes of squamous cells

   D **False**   cytological washings may demonstrate hyphae

   E **False**   Radiology occasionally reveals a shaggy mucosa and in some cases stricture formation. However, endoscopy is the best method of detecting and confirming *moniliasis*

                                    Cecil, p. 631
                             Brocklehurst, p. 510–511

5.32 The following is/are true

A   in type A *gastritis* the antrum is primarily involved
B   90 per cent of patients with pernicious anaemia have parietal cell antibodies
C   parietal cell antibodies are usually associated with type B gastritis
D   pepsin secretion is decreased in chronic gastritis
E   when gastritis involves the antrum serum gastin levels are elevated

5.33 *Menetrière's disease* is characterised by

A   hypersecretion of gastric acid
B   gastric mucosal hypertrophy
C   hypoproteinaemia
D   weight loss
E   nausea and vomiting

5.34 The following is/are true of *gastric ulcers*

A   they occur frequently in the elderly
B   chronic gastritis is present in almost all patients with chronic gastric ulcer
C   one third of all deaths due to gastric ulcer occur in the elderly
D   there is a significant correlation between ulcer size and duration of symptoms
E   intestinal metaplasia is a commonly associated feature

(Answers overleaf)

5.32 A **False**   *chronic gastritis* is divided into type A and type B
depending on the anatomical portion of the stomach
involved and the presence or absence of parietal cell
antibodies. Type A involves the body and fundus of
the stomach and parietal cell antibodies and
pernicious anaemia are associated. Type B involves
the antrum, parietal cell antibodies do not occur but
antibodies to gastrin producing cells have recently
been found
   B **True**
   C **False**
   D **True**   gastric acid secretion and pepsin secretion are
decreased in chronic gastritis
   E **False**   in *type A gastritis* there is hypo or achlorhydria and
elevated serum gastrin concentrations. In *type B
gastritis*, acid secretion is usually diminished and
gastrin levels are within the normal range
                                                    Cecil, p. 634

5.33 A **False**   hyposecretion of gastric acid
   B **True**   gastric mucosal hypertrophy with giant ruggae
   C **True**   there is increased loss of protein from the stomach
with weight loss and oedema
   D **True**
   E **True**   patients may present with pain, nausea and vomiting
                                                    Cecil, p. 634
                                            Brocklehurst, p. 518

5.34 A **True**   autopsy data report figures from 5.2 per cent for
patients over 65 years of age to 8.5 per cent in the over
70 age group
   B **True**   in patients with *duodenal ulcer*, the *gastritis* is limited
to the pyloric area and is mild. *Gastric ulcers* almost
always occur in mucosa involved by gastritis
   C **True**
   D **True**   the largest ulcers occur in patients with the longest
duration of symptoms
   E **False**
                                            Brocklehurst, pp 514–515

5.35 The following is/are true of the _bile acid breath test_

A   it is useful in the diagnosis of small bowel bacterial overgrowth

B   it is characterised by excessive large bowel absorption of ^{14}C glycine-cholate

C   it is characterised by excessive $^{14}CO_2$ excretion in the breath

D   it is a more accurate diagnostic test of bacterial overgrowth than measurement of urinary indican excretion

E   breath measurements are taken half an hour after bile salt ingestion

5.36 The following is/are true

A   the upper small intestine is bacteria free in all normal subjects

B   the terminal ileum has concentrations of organisms approaching 10^5 to 10^8 per g

C   bacteroides are rarely cultured in the colon

D 10^4 organisms per ml of jejunal aspirate is abnormal

E   elevated urinary 5-hydroxyindole-acetic acid is supportive evidence of bacterial overgrowth

5.37 Diverticuli in the duodenum

A   occur with increasing frequency in the elderly

B   may present with diarrhoea

C   are frequently multiple

D   are always associated with bacterial overgrowth

E   are frequently associated with low levels of iron, folate and vitamin B12

(Answers overleaf)

5.35 A **True**   it is helpful in the diagnosis of malabsorption caused by disorders in which bile acid deconjugation is abnormal. These include *bacterial overgrowth* in the small intestine and the terminal ileum (which impair reabsorption of bile salts and therefore increase their loss into the colon)

B **False**   small intestinal bacteria deconjugate a significant amount of orally administered ^{14}CO glycine-cholate before it is absorbed

C **True**   released ^{14}C glycine will be further metabolised by bacterial enzymes to $^{14}CO_2$, which quickly diffuses into the circulation and can be measured in expired air

D **True**   *urinary indican* and *5 hydroxyindole-acetic acid [5 HIAA)* are elevated in diseases of ileal dysfunction and adult *coeliac disease* as well as diseases of bacterial overgrowth

E **False**   when significant bacterial overgrowth is present, $^{14}CO_2$ *excretion* in the breath is elevated ten-fold at 4 to 5 hours

Cecil, pp 686–687

5.36 A **False**   the upper small intestine is bacteria free in one-third of normal subjects; in the remainder, gram positive or facultative anaerobes are present (lactobacilli and enterococci) in concentrations of 10^1 to 10^3 organisms per gram of content. Coliforms may be transiently present but rarely exceed 10^3 per g

B **True**
C **False**   in the colon enormous concentrations of anaerobes — bacteroides, lactobacilli and clostridia — are usually present

D **True**
E **True**

Cecil, p 687
McEvoy, British Medical Journal 1983

5.37 A **True**   diverticuli in the duodenum occur with increasing frequency in the elderly, being rare before the age of 40

B **True**   the symptomatology is varied and may include diarrhoea, dyspepsia, anaemia, weight loss or mental confusion

C **True**
D **False**   but they may be associated with bacterial overgrowth and hence malabsorption syndromes

E **True**

Brocklehurst, pp 518–519

5.38 *Villous atrophy* **is found in**
  A   adult coeliac disease
  B   small bowel lymphoma
  C   Whipple's disease
  D   giardiosis
  E   Crohn's disease

5.39 **Chronic** *small bowel ischaemia*
  A   is caused by atherosclerosis of the coeliac artery
  B   may cause malabsorption
  C   has classical histological changes
  D   is associated with polyarteritis nodosa
  E   occurs in Degos' disease

5.40 **The following is/are true of malignant** *small bowel tumours*
  A   primary lymphoma is the most frequently
       diagnosed malignancy
  B   small bowel tumours account for less than 5 per cent of all
       bowel tumours
  C   the majority occur in patients over 50 years old
  D   adenocarcinoma usually occurs in the lower small intestine
  E   over 10 per cent of patients with adult coeliac disease
       develop small bowel lymphoma

(Answers overleaf)

5.38 A **True**   gluten sensitive *villous atrophy*
     B **True**   non-gluten sensitive villous atrophy. This may present
                   with a small bowel malabsorption syndrome which is
                   clinically and radiologically indentical to adult coeliac
                   disease
     C **True**   the diagnosis of *Whipple's* disease depends on the
                   finding of periodic acid — Schiff (PAS) positive
                   macrophages infiltrating involved tissues
     D **True**
     E **Falşe**

                                            Cecil, pp 688, 695–696

5.39 A **True**   chronic ischaemia of the small bowel is usually
                   caused by atherosclerosis of the superior and
                   inferior coeliac arteries
     B **True**   presumably because of impaired mucosal cell
                   function
     C **False**   no classical histological changes have been
                   demonstrated in chronic *small bowel ischaemia*
                   associated with *malabsorption*
     D **True**
     E **True**   *Degos' disease* is characterised by necrotic skin
                   lesions and vasculitis of the small gut. It may also
                   cause malabsorption, although the far more serious
                   and common clinical manifestation is infarction of the
                   gut

                                                        Cecil, p. 697

5.40 A **False**   adenocarcinoma is the most frequent
     B **True**
     C **True**
     D **False**   most occur in the upper small intestine within 25 cm
                   of the ligament of Treitz
     E **True**   it is believed that lymphoma is more common in those
                   not treated with a gluten free diet. Relapse in patients
                   who have responded to a gluten free diet should alert
                   one to the possibility of a small bowel lymphoma

                                            Platt, pp 21–22
                                            Cecil, pp 698–699

5.41   *Chronic pancreatitis*

A   is seen in younger rather than older patients
B   is associated with radiographic calcification in one-third of patients
C   may be relapsing
D   is associated with alcoholism and cholelithiasis
E   rarely presents with pancreatic insufficiency

5.42   An elderly female presents for the first time with bright red rectal bleeding from *diverticular disease*. The following is/are true

A   haemorrhage always occurs in inflamed diverticulae
B   bleeding usually stops spontaneously
C   the left colon is the commonest site of bleeding
D   the incidence of rebleeding is low
E   elective surgery is usually indicated

(Answers overleaf)

5.41 A **False**   since *pancreatic insufficiency* takes many years to develop, it is seen in older, rather than younger patients

     B **True**

     C **True**   *chronic pancreatitis* may be relapsing, in which case there are repeated acute attacks; it may present with chronic pain, or with little or no early symptoms, so that the initial manifestations are related to the maldigestion of pancreatic enzyme insufficiency

     D **True**   it is also associated with hyperparathyroidism, trauma, malnutrition and steroids

     E **False**

Platt, p. 25

5.42 A **False**   haemorrhage may occur from uninflamed diverticulae. Intramural arterial branches run in close proximity to the nect and dome of the out-pouching. Initial thickening and eccentric rupture of these branches on the side of the vessel facing the bowel lumen have been described

     B **True**

     C **False**   bleeding more commonly results from the right than from the left colon

     D **True**   if bleeding does stop spontaneously the incidence of rebleeding is low, therefore elective surgery is not indicated after the first bleeding episode

     E **False**   depending on the clinical situation elective surgery should be considered after the second or third episode. Prior to surgery the site of bleeding should be localised by selective abdominal angiography. Bleeding from a diverticulum must be differentiated from bleeding from angiodysplasia of the caecum or right colon since the latter usually require a more limited resection

Platt, pp 33–34

5.43   In *ischaemic colitis*

A   pain begins suddenly
B   symptoms are initially out of proportion to physical findings
C   peritonitis rarely develops
D   angiography is the investigation of choice
E   submucosal haemorrhage can be identified at endoscopy

5.44   *Pseudomembranous colitis* occurs as a complication of

A   antibiotic therapy
B   uraemia
C   intestinal ischaemia
D   inflammatory bowel disease
E   intestinal obstruction

5.45   *Colorectal cancer*

A   is the most common gastrointestinal cancer
B   is an adenocarcinoma in over 94 per cent of cases
C   is more common in males
D   incidence rates decrease with age over 45 years
E   develops in over 20 per cent of patients with ulcerative
     colitis for 25 years or more

**5.46   *Carcinoembryonic antigen* in the serum of patients with
         colorectal cancer**

A   reflects tumour bulk
B   is useful for detection of recurrence after surgery
C   is useful in screening for tumour
D   is useful for detection of metastatic disease after surgery
E   is a glycoprotein

(Answers overleaf)

5.43 A **True**   pain is severe and begins suddenly
     B **True**   an important clue to the presence of *ischaemic colitis*
                   and other vascular syndromes is that, at least initially,
                   the severity of pain is usually out of proportion to the
                   physical findings
     C **False**   with *bowel infarction*, the signs of an acute surgical
                   abdomen and peritonitis develop within a few hours
     D **False**   *angiography* may sometimes be helpful, but
                   frequently will be normal. If the patient's clinical
                   condition permits, barium enema can be performed. A
                   characteristic *thumb printing* pattern, due to
                   submucosal haemorrhage, is often present
     E **True**

                                        Brocklehurst, pp 546–548
                                            Cecil, pp 721–722
                                                Platt, p. 35

5.44 A **True**   the commonest cause is, of course, antibiotic therapy.
     B **True**   Occasionally it may occur in healthy persons with no
     C **True**   identifiable cause. There is an increased risk of
     D **True**   developing antibiotic associated *pseudomembranous*
     E **True**   *colitis* with increasing age

                                             Cecil, p. 1497
                                            Platt, pp 36–37

5.45 A **True**
     B **True**
     C **False**   *colonic cancer* involves both sexes at similar rates
     D **False**   the age specific incidence rates rise steadily until age
                   85, after which a slight drop off is noted probably
                   because of incomplete case findings in the very old
     E **True**   with less than a decade of disease the carcinoma risk
                   is small, rising to a cumulative incidence of 25–40 per
                   cent at 25 years

                                            Platt, pp 38–40

5.46 A **True**
     B **True**
     C **False**   it is positive in 60–90 per cent of patients with colonic
                   cancer depending on (a) extent of the disease; (b) type
                   of the tumour, i.e. anaplastic lesions have a lower
                   incidence; (c) the presence or absence of liver
                   metastases. The onset of hepatic involvement with
                   tumour is often heralded by a sharp increase in
                   carcinoembryonic antigen levels
     D **True**
     E **True**   with a molecular weight of 200 000 daltons

                                            Platt, pp 40–41
                                             Cecil, p. 1021

5.47 _Volvulus_ of the colon

   A   occurs predominantly in middle age
   B   is common in Africa
   C   is associated with hypocalcaemia
   D   rarely requires operative intervention
   E   is associated with Parkinsonism

5.48 _Idiopathic megacolon_

   A   complicates constipation in the elderly
   B   presents as gross abdominal tympanic distention
   C   is associated with diarrhoea and faecal incontinence
   D   is best diagnosed by barium studies
   E   may develop into a sigmoid volvulus

5.49 _Gastro-oesophageal reflux_ may be induced by which of the following

   A   smoking
   B   metoclopromide
   C   gastrin
   D   Bethanechol
   E   anticholinergic drugs

5.50 An elderly man who does not drink alcohol presents with an episode of _acute pancreatitis_. Which of the following might have caused this episode

   A   diabetic ketoacidosis
   B   hyperparathyroidism
   C   thiazide diuretics
   D   azothioprine
   E   hyperlipoproteinaemia

(Answers overleaf)

5.47 A **False**   the mean age of onset is 65 years. It occurs
particularly in institutionalised and immobile patients
from mental hospitals. 50 per cent of cases are over 70
years
   B **True**   the disorder is more common in Africa than the
United Kingdom where it is associated with a high
residue diet
   C **False**   it is associated with hypercalcaemia, explosive
treatment of constipation, and high residue diet
   D **False**   sigmoidoscopy is all that is required in some cases
but over 50 per cent require operative intervention
   E **True**   this may be due to the use of anticholinergic drugs
although the exact mechanism of altered bowel
motility in Parkinsonism has not yet been established
                                        Brocklehurst, pp 538–539

5.48 A **True**   *faecal incontinence* and idiopathic *megacolon* are two
important complications of *constipation* in the elderly
   B **True**
   C **True**
   D **False**   the diagnosis is easily made by plain abdominal films.
Often, these frail patients would not withstand a
barium enema
   E **True**   this is the main danger of idiopathic megacolon
                                        Brocklehurst, p. 538

5.49 A **True**   smoking and anticholinergic drugs both decrease
lower oesophageal sphincter pressure
   B **False**   metoclopromide, gastrin and bethanecol all increase
lower *oesophageal sphincter* pressure
   C **False**
   D **False**
   E **True**
                                        Cecil, p. 626

5.50 A **False**   raised glucose levels are associated with pancreatitis;
diabetic ketoacidosis is associated with elevated
serum amylase levels but not with acute pancreatitis
   B **True**
   C **True**
   D **True**   isoniazid, steroids, oral contraceptives and methyl
alcohol have all been implicated
   E **False**   type I, IV and V are associated with pancreatitis but
would be most unlikely causes in an elderly man
                                        Cecil, pp 733–734

5.51 *Angiodysplasia* **of the large bowel is characterised by**

A   specific appearances on mesenteric angiography
B   lesions visible at laparotomy
C   reliable diagnosis on barium enema
D   presentation before middle age
E   lesions present in the descending colon

5.52 **The following is/are true of** *angiodysplasia*

A   iron deficiency anaemia is rare
B   barium studies are normal
C   the diagnosis is best made by superior mesenteric angiography
D   early venous filling is seen radiographically
E   lesions characteristically occur in the sigmoid colon

(Answers overleaf)

5.51 A **True**
      B **False**
      C **False**
      D **False**   the characteristic picture is that of an elderly person
                      presenting with an *iron deficiency anaemia*, normal
                      barium meal and enema and positive occult blood in
                      the stool
      E **False**   lesions are mainly seen in the caecum and ascending
                      colon

                                          Cecil, pp 816-817

5.52 A **False**   characteristically patients are elderly, presenting with
                      an *iron deficiency anaemia*, normal barium studies,
                      and positive tests for faecal occult blood loss
      B **True**
      C **True**
      D **True**   characteristically, angiographic changes are of
                      multiple small arteriovenous filling abnormalities and
                      early venous filling
      E **False**

                                          Cecil, p. 817
                                          Platt, p. 36

6. Haematology

6.1 The following is/are true of *iron deficiency* anaemia in the elderly

A an *oesophageal web* commonly occurs
B a superficial gastritis appears early
C gastric atrophy may occur
D gastric parietal cell antibodies are commonly found
E iron absorption is decreased

6.2 Iron absorption

A is independent of body iron stores
B is increased in iron deficiency anaemia
C is increased in *haemochramosis*
D is assisted by hydrochloric acid
E is better from meat than from vegetable sources

6.3 The following characteristically cause *hypochromic anaemia*

A chronic infection
B acute haemorrhage
C uraemia
D protein deficiency
E thalassaemia

6.4 The following cause *macrocytosis*

A haemolysis
B aplastic anaemia
C alcohol ingestion
D cirrhosis
E sideroblastic anaemia

(Answers overleaf)

6.1 A **False**   an *oesophageal web* is rare; it is premalignant
     B **True**   a *superficial gastritis* appears early and acid secretion
                     diminishes; as *atrophic gastritis* develops the cellular
                     infiltration decreases and acid secretion falls; the final
                     picture of *gastric atrophy* is identical with that seen in
                     pernicious anaemia
     C **True**
     D **True**   *gastric parietal cell antibodies* are commonly found in
                     patients with iron deficiency *anaemia* and histamine
                     fast achlorhydria and their prevalence increases with
                     age
     E **False**

                                                    Brocklehurst, pp 849–855

6.2 A **False**   *iron* absorption varies with body iron stores
     B **True**
     C **False**   iron absorption is decreased in states of overload,
                     with the exception of *haemochromatosis*
     D **True**   it is also increased by *ascorbic acid*
     E **True**   there is a marked variation in absorption of iron from
                     food stuffs. Absorption is much better from muscle
                     and haemoglobin than from vegetable sources and
                     eggs

                                                    Brocklehurst, p. 850

6.3 A **True**
     B **False**   characteristically causes a *macrocytic anaemia* due to
                     the increase in circulating reticulocytes
     C **True**   although the anaemia associated with uraemia it is
                     often normochromic
     D **False**   causes a macrocytic anaemia
     E **True**

hypochromic anaemia is also associated with *sideroblastic
anaemia, infection, rheumatoid arthritis* and malignancy, but the
commonest cause in the elderly is chronic gastrointestinal blood
loss

                                                    Cecil, pp 851–853
                                                    Brocklehurst, p. 885

6.4 A **True**
     B **True**
     C **True**
     D **True**
     E **True**

Other causes are *haemorrhage, leukaemia, marrow infiltration or
replacement, myxoedema, hypopituitarism, protein deficiency* and
scurvy

                                                    Cecil, pp 801, 843, 852, 1371

6.5   Vitamin B12 deficiency occurs in

A   ileal resection
B   ileal tuberculosis
C   phytate ingestion
D   *blind loop syndrome*
E   villous adenoma

6.6   *Eosinophilia* is characteristically associated with

A   psoriasis
B   post splenectomy
C   atopic eczema
D   pemphigus
E   polyarteritis nodosa

6.7   *Plasma cell reactions* may occur in

A   chronic infection
B   metastatic disease
C   rheumatoid arthritis
D   hydronephrosis
E   chronic liver disease

6.8   In *benign monoclonal gammopathy*

A   the IgG level does not exceed 5 g/dl
B   the immunoglobulin level gradually rises over a follow up period
C   the marrow contains less than 9 per cent plasma cells
D   Bence Jones proteinuria is common
E   other serum immunoglobulin levels are not depressed

(Answers overleaf)

6.5 A **True**   any ileal lesions such as resection, *tuberculosis,*
                    Crohn's, or *ulcerative colitis* may lead to *vitamin B12*
                    deficiency

     B **True**
     C **True**   chelating agents such as phytates may lead to vitamin
                    B12 deficiency
     D **True**   B12 utilisation by bacteria in blind loop syndrome and
                    jejunal diverticulosis leads to deficiency
     E **False**   *villous adenomas* present with watery diarrhoea,
                    hypokalaemia, mucous discharge and occasionally a
                    protein losing enteropathy

                                          Brocklehurst, pp 861–863

6.6 A **False**
     B **True**
     C **True**
     D **False**
     E **True**

eosinophilia is also associated with *food allergies, parasites,
scabies, dermatitis herpiformis, asthma, Loeffler's syndrome,*
rebound post-infections, *blood dyscrasias, Hodgkin's disease,* and
rheumatoid arthritis

                                          Cecil, pp 375–376

6.7 A **True**
     B **True**
     C **True**
     D **False**   hydronephrosis is associated with secondary
                    polycythaemia
     E **True**

                                          Cecil, pp 963–972

6.8 A **False**   the IgG level should not exceed 2 g/dl
     B **False**   the level should remain steady or fall, but not rise
     C **True**
     D **False**   there should be no Bence Jones proteinuria
     E **True**

All of the above factors are necessary to make a diagnosis of
benign monoclonal gammopathy but patients in whom the
diagnosis is made do require follow-up; in some cases multiple
myeloma may remain in such a phase for many years before overt
signs appear

                                          Brocklehurst, p. 876

6.9   *Multiple myeloma* is characterised by

A   raised serum calcium levels
B   normal serum phosphate levels
C   raised serum *alkaline phosphatase* levels
D   osteosclerotic lesions
E   *hyperuricaemia*

6.10   The following is/are true of *multiple myeloma*

A   skeletal radiographic changes are absent in up to 10 per cent of cases
B   urinary light chains flocculate when heated slowly between 50 and 60 degrees centigrade
C   anaemia of some degree almost invariably occurs
D   all immunoglobin levels are elevated
E   renal insufficiency is rare

6.11   Osteolytic lesions occur in the following

A   metastatic thyroid carcinoma
B   multiple myeloma
C   malignant carcinoid
D   Hodgkin's disease
E   renal neoplasm

(Answers overleaf)

6.9 A **True**
   B **True** unless there is associated renal failure in which case levels rise
   C **False** the alkaline phosphatase is normal or only slightly raised, a point of major importance in the differential diagnosis of *multiple myeloma, hyperparathyroidism* and secondary carcinoma of bone in which significant elevation is usual
   D **False** bone changes consist of diffuse decalcification or localised areas of bone destruction (*osteolytic* lesions) or a combination of both. The localised lesions appear as rounded discrete punched-out areas with no sclerosis at the margin. They occur in bones normally containing red marrow, and are especially common in the skull
   E **True**

de Gruchy, pp 533–540

6.10 A **True** thus the absence of skeletal radiographic changes does not necessarily exclude the diagnosis
   B **True** the *Bence Jones protein* dissolves on boiling and reappears on cooling below 60°C
   C **True**
   D **False** normal *immunoglobulins* are depressed
   E **False** Chronic renal insufficiency frequently develops during the course of the disease and occasionally is an initial manifestation. In the absence of coexistent essential hypertension the blood pressure is normal. For this reason myeloma should be considered as a probable cause in any patient with chronic renal insufficiency and a normal blood pressure

de Gruchy, pp 533–540

6.11 A **True**
   B **True**
   C **False** *osteosclerotic* lesions are associated with both malignant *carcinoid* and *Hodgkin's* disease
   D **False**
   E **True**
Other causes of *osteolytic* lesions are renal and lower bowel neoplasms and *malignant lymphoma. Prostatic and breast neoplasms* are associated with either osteolytic or osteosclerotic lesions

Cecil, p. 696

6.12 *Secondary polycythemia* **is characteristically associated with**

    A   sulphaemoglobinaemia
    B   hydronephrosis
    C   myeloproliferative disorders
    D   *Hodgkin's disease*
    E   uterine myomata

6.13 *Thrombocytopenia* **may be caused by**

    A   uraemia
    B   thiazide diuretics
    C   haemorrhage
    D   polycythemia rubra vera
    E   alcoholism

6.14 *Platelet dysfunction* **is associated with**

    A   Aspirin ingestion
    B   scurvy
    C   dysproteinaemia
    D   uraemia
    E   thrombocythaemia

6.15 **The following drugs may cause** *leukocytosis*

    A   aspirin
    B   steroids
    C   digitalis
    D   thiouracil
    E   adrenaline

(Answers overleaf)

6.12 A **True**   it is also associated with *methaemoglobinaemia*
    B **True**   *hypernephroma, polycystic kidney* disease, *renal artery stenosis*, and renal transplantation are also associated
    C **False**   *polycythaemia rubra vera* is associated with myeloproliferative disorders
    D **False**
    E **True**

There are a number of other disorders associated with *secondary polycythaemia*: any cause of *hypoxia, carcinoma of liver, cerebellar haemangioblastoma, virilising syndromes, phaeochromocytoma, haemoglobinopathies,* hypertransfusion, dehydration and *Gaisboch's syndrome* (hypertension, anxiety, high normal red cell mass and low normal plama volume).

de Gruchy, pp 555–560

6.13 A **True**
    B **True**   also sulphonamides, quinine, rifampicin, and nonsteroidal anti-inflammatory drugs, and many other agents
    C **True**
    D **False**   thrombocytosis is associated with polycythaemia rubra vera
    E **True**

de Gruchy, p. 650

6.14 A **True**   also with indomethacin, phenylbutazone and dextran infusions
    B **True**
    C **True**
    D **True**
    E **True**   any of the myeloproliferative disorders can be associated with *platelet dysfunction*

de Gruchy, pp 673–675

6.15 A **False**   results in qualitative platelet defects
    B **True**
    C **True**
    D **False**   causes a selective *neutropenia*
    E **True**

de Gruchy, pp 396–398

6.16   The following may be associated with *lymphocytosis*

A   polyarteritis nodosa
B   tuberculosis
C   dermatitis herpetiformis
D   thyrotoxicosis
E   myelomatosis

6.17   The following may cause *thrombocytosis*

A   haemorrhage
B   treatment of pernicious anaemia
C   disseminated intravascular coagulation
D   chronic renal failure
E   alcohol

6.18   The following is/are true of *senile* (involutional) *purpura*

A   petechiae are more commonly found than purpuric lesions
B   lesions mainly occur on the neck and trunk
C   the tourniquet test is usually positive
D   histological section of the skin in affected areas shows marked atrophy of collagen
E   lesions persist for a long period

(Answers overleaf)

6.16 A **False**   associated with an *eosinophilia*
     B **True**   and also causes *monocytosis*
     C **False**   causes eosinophilia
     D **True**
     E **True**

Other causes are *viral infections*, convalescence from acute *bacterial infections, syphilis, brucellosis, toxoplasmosis, myaesthenia gravis*, and carcinoma

de Gruchy, pp 402–403 1

6.17 A **True**   *haemorrhage* may initially be associated with *thrombocytopaenia*
     B **True**   rebound *thrombocytosis* may occur after treatment of *pernicious anaemia* and after recovery from haemolysis
     C **False**   thrombocytopaenia
     D **True**   chronic *renal failure* may also be associated with qualitative platelet defects and thrombocytopaenia
     E **False**   thrombocytopaenia

Other disease states associated with the thrombocytosis are *malignancy, myeloproliferative disorders*, and chronic inflammatory disease.

de Gruchy, pp 675–676

6.18 A **False**   it is characterised by purpuric areas which are large, irregular, dark purple and have a clear cut margin. The skin in affected areas is inelastic, thin, smooth, pigmented and may show non-pigmented areas
     B **False**   lesions occur on the extensor surface and radial border of the forearm and on the back of the hand. They do not extend to the fingers and generally do not occur in other parts of the body
     C **False**   the *tourniquet test* is negative
     D **True**
     E **True**   because of collagen atrophy the skin is freely mobile over deeper tissues. Purpuric lesions are induced by sheering strain to the skin which tears the vessels and abnormally extensive spread of blood is allowed by the atrophied collagen fibres. *The lesions persist for long periods because of slow* resorption of blood by impaired phagocytosis

de Gruchy, pp 633, 634

6.19   The following is/are associated with *leuco-erythroblastic anaemia*

  A   prostatic skeletal metastases
  B   primary sideroblastic anaemia
  C   multiple myeloma
  D   myelosclerosis
  E   malignant lymphomas

6.20   The following may cause a secondary *sideroblastic anaemia*

  A   alcohol
  B   lead
  C   isoniazid
  D   nutritional *megaloblastic anaemia*
  E   myeloproliferative disorders

6.21   The following is/are true of primary *sideroblastic anaemia*

  A   a moderately enlarged spleen is usually present
  B   serum iron levels are low
  C   the percentage saturation of iron binding protein is normal
  D   the bone marrow is hyperplastic
  E   erythropoeisis shows a shift to the right

(Answers overleaf)

6.19 A **True**   secondary carcinoma of bone is the commonest cause
     B **False**
     C **True**
     D **True**
     E **True**
Leuco-erythroblastic anaemia results from infiltration of bone by
foreign or abnormal tissue and it is characterised by immature
myeloid and nucleated red blood cells in the peripheral blood
film. Other causes not encountered in elderly patients are the
lipoid dystrophies and marble bone disease

de Gruchy, pp 490–491

6.20 A **True**   other causes of *sideroblastic anaemia* are *cycloserine,*
     B **True**   *chloramphenicol, haemolytic anaemia*, infections,
     C **True**   *collagen vascular diseases*, erythroleukaemia, other
     D **True**   acute non-lymphoblastic *leukaemias* and cutaneous
     E **True**   *porphyria*

de Gruchy, p. 116
Burton, p. 77

6.21 A **False**   the *spleen* is either not palpable or just palpable
                    below the costal margin
     B **False**   serum iron is normal or moderately raised
     C **True**   the percentage saturation of iron-binding protein is
                    normal or only slightly increased
     D **True**   mainly due to erythroid hyperplasia
     E **False**   erythropoeisis is usually normoblastic but commonly
                    macronormoblastic. Erythropoeisis shows a shift to
                    the left and late normoblasts often have vacuolated
                    cytoplasm
Primary *sideroblastic anaemia* occurs mainly in middle-aged and
elderly subjects. The features are a moderately severe anaemia
with dimorphic red blood cells, a normal or raised serum iron and
normal or raised iron binding capacity. The marrow has
increased iron stores — a greater number and size of iron
granules. The iron granules may form a peripheral ring in the
cytoplasm of some marrow cells — ring sideroblasts.

de Gruchy, pp 116–117

6.22   The following is/are characteristically associated with
**   *myeloclerosis***

- A   a previous diagnosis of polycythemia rubra vera
- B   splenic infarction
- C   leucoerythroblastic anaemia
- D   tear and pear shaped poikilocytosis
- E   anaemia

6.23   *Myeloclerosis* is characteristically associated with

- A   jaundice
- B   epigastric discomfort
- C   purpura
- D   hyperuricaemia
- E   thrombocytopenia

(Answers overleaf)

6.22 A **True**
B **True**   the *spleen* is frequently grossly enlarged; splenic infarcts commonly occur. Hepatic enlargement is also present
C **True**
D **True**
E **True**   anaemia is almost invariably present but its severity and rate of progress vary considerably. Impaired red cell production, haemolysis and increased plasma volume associated with splenomegaly all contribute to the anaemia. Characteristically the blood film shows marked *anisocytosis* and *poikilocytosis* with tear-shaped poikilocytes.

de Gruchy, pp 585–588

6.23 A **True**   *hepatomegaly* is common and associated with mild jaundice
B **True**   because of *splenomegaly*, epigastric discomfort after meals, nausea, flatulence and left hypochondrial fullness occur
C **True**   Bleeding manifestations are usually due to *thrombocytopenia*
D **True**   gout is a common complication
E **True**

de Gruchy, pp 585, 588

7. Immunology and microbiology

7.1 The following is/are true

A   IgG antibody is associated with the primary immune response

B   antigenic memory is retained by T lymphocytes

C   IgM antibody is associated with the secondary immune response

D   all antigens are taken up by macrophages

E   B lymphocytes form plasma cells

7.2 Immunoglobulins

A   are serum proteins

B   contain four polypeptide chains

C   have constant amino terminal amino acid sequences

D   have carboxy terminal ends which contain the antigen binding site

E   are antigen specific single molecules

7.3 The following is/are true of immunoglobulins

A   IgG is a dimer

B   IgA is found in respiratory secretions

C   IgA contains an additional secretory protein

D   IgM is mostly found in gastric secretions

E   IgE binds to mast cells

(Answers overleaf)

7.1 A **False**   an *immune response* which results from first contact
with an antigen is known as the primary response.
Antibody appears in the serum 10–20 days after
contact. The antibody is IgM
   B **False**   after the primary response, antibody disappears but
memory of the event is retained by sensitised
B *lymphocytes*
   C **False**   subsequent exposure to the same antigen results in a
secondary response with IgG production after a
period of 5–7 days
   D **True**   the macrophages then interact with lymphocytes
   E **True**   *plasma cells* produce specific antibody of the IgM
class

Brocklehurst, pp 82–83

7.2 A **True**
   B **True**   *immunoglobulins* contain two polypeptide heavy
chains and two polypeptide light chains
   C **False**   the carboxy terminal portions of both heavy and light
chains contain a constant region where amino acid
sequences are invariable. Alternatively, the amino
terminal contains highly variable sequences of amino
acids and contains the antigen binding site
   D **False**
   E **True**   a single molecule has a fixed amino acid sequence
and is antigen specific

Brocklehurst, pp 83–84

7.3 A **False**   IgG is the major immunoglobulin in the serum and
exists as a monomer
   B **True**   it is the major immunoglobulin in mucosal secretions
and exists as a dimer. It has additional protein known
as the secretory protein which allows transport across
epithelium and aids in resisting enzymic degradation
   C **True**
   D **False**   IgM is largely confined to serum and exists as a
pentamer
   E **True**   and is involved in immediate hypersensitivity
reactions

Brocklehurst, pp 83–84

7.4   The following factors change with increasing age

A   circulating *lymphocyte* numbers
B   T *lymphocyte* function
C   contact sensitivity to *dinitrochlorobenzene*
D   delayed hypersensitivity reaction to tuberculin
E   levels of natural antibody

7.5   The following is/are true

A   *neutrophil* numbers reduce with ageing
B   neutrophils are attracted to sites of infection by antibody
C   chemotaxis is impaired in the majority of elderly
D   lactoferrin is a bactericidal enzyme
E   neutrophils activate the complement system

7.6   The following increase with age

A   *antibody* production
B   autoantibodies
C   autoimmune diseases
D   pernicious anaemia
E   idiopathic hypothyroidism

7.7   In an elderly stroke patient with previous *ischaemic heart disease* chest infection may present as

A   urinary incontinence
B   falls
C   a lower level of functional capacity for rehabilitation
D   exacerbation of ischaemic symptoms
E   faecal incontinence

(Answers overleaf)

7.4 A **False** circulating *lymphocyte* numbers do not change with age

    B **True**
    C **True**
    D **True**
    E **True** *antibody* production is impaired in both primary and secondary responses probably due to thymic involution and reduced T helper lymphocyte function

7.5 A **True** the normal range for the total *leucocyte count* in old age is 3000–8500 per mm^3 (3.0–8.5 × 10^9/l) (from a large community survey of old people). Leucocyte counts do show a tendency to leucopenia
    B **False** *neutrophils* are attracted to infection or injury by chemotactic factors
    C **False** chemotaxis is intact in the majority of elderly studied
    D **True** bactericidal enzymes are contained in the cytoplasmic granules of neutrophils and include lysozyme, myeloperoxidase, hydrolases and lactoferrin
    E **False** *bacteria* directly activate the complement system; chemotactic factor, which attracts neutrophils, is a product of this activation

Brocklehurst, pp 87–88

7.6 A **False** *antibody* production declines probably due to thymic involution and reduced T helper lymphocyte function
    B **True** antibodies to nuclear antigens, immunoglobulins (rheumatoid factor), gastric parietal cell and thyroid increase in frequency with advancing age
    C **False** autoimmune disease does not increase in frequency with age
    D **True**
    E **True**

Brocklehurst, pp 87–88

7.7 A **True**
    B **True**
    C **True**
    D **True**
    E **True** due to faecal impaction and spurious diarrhoea.
With advancing age there is an increased incidence of 'silent presentation' — the damping down of characteristic responses. Therefore, illness of any form may present as urinary or faecal *incontinence,* instability or *falling,, immobility* and *confusion*; these are known as the Geriatric Giants.

Brocklehurst, pp 92–93

7.8 *Hospital acquired infections* **increase in frequency in**
   A   the elderly
   B   malnutrition
   C   diabetic ketoacidosis
   D   uraemia
   E   the use of urinary catheters

7.9 **The following is/are true of** *septicaemia*
   A   it describes the temporary presence of bacteria in the blood
   B   the incidence is increasing
   C   endotoxins are released by pneumococcus
   D   fever is often absent in the elderly
   E   the majority of positive cultures are obtained from third and
       fourth blood cultures

7.10 **The following is/are true of** *pneumococcus*
   A   its prevalence increases with age
   B   capsular polysaccharide enhances phagocytosis
   C   over 80 capsular antigens have been defined
   D   annual vaccination is necessary for immunisation
   E   pneumococcal vaccine is strongly recommended for
       institutionalised elderly

(Answers overleaf)

7.8 A **True**   the most common infections are urinary tract, surgical wounds, pneumonia and bacteraemia
B **True**   malnutrition is not uncommon in the hospitalised elderly
C **True**
D **True**   Both diabetic ketoacidosis and uraemia give rise to impaired defence mechanisms and particularly affect polymorphonuclear phagocytic function
E **True**   *Escherischia coli* and proteus are the common organisms

Brocklehurst, p. 93

7.9 A **False**   *bacteraemia* describes the temporary presence of bacteria in the blood without the establishment of a general infection and with no response from the host. Alternatively, *septicaemia* implies the persistent presence of bacteria which multiply and produce illness
B **True**   presumably related to modern technological medicine
C **False**   *endotoxins* are released by gram-negative organisms, *exotoxins* by gram-positive organisms such as *pneumococci*
D **True**   the onset is atypical — classical signs and symptoms may be absent, i.e. confusion is more prominent and fever often absent
E **False**   most positive results are obtained from the first two cultures. If infection is defined as a problem in the elderly, 10 per cent of blood cultures will yield positive and meaningful results

Brocklehurst, pp 94–95

7.10 A **True**   the prevalence increases dramatically with age
B **False**   the organism is successful in host invasion because of its capsule; the polysaccharide inhibits phagocytosis
C **True**   currently available vaccines contain approximately 14 capsular antigens
D **False**   protective levels of antibody persist for 5 to 8 years; thus revaccination is not required for at least 5 years
E **False**   there is increasing evidence of side-effects with advancing age in up to 60 per cent of older people and vaccination is of no proven value in the institutionalised elderly

Brocklehurst, p. 97

7.11   The following is/are true of *influenza*

A   the over 65s account for 10 per cent of cases
B   there is extensive cross reactivity between viral subtypes
C   Serum antibody response begins within 24 h of initial influenza vaccine
D   immunisation against influenza is ineffective in the elderly
E   immunisation should be repeated at 5 yearly intervals

7.12   The following are causative organisms in gram — negative *septic shock*

A   Bacteroides
B   Clostridia
C   Klebsiella-Enterobacter
D   Streptococcus
E   Serratia

7.13   Late stages of *septic shock* are characterised by

A   high cardiac output
B   metabolic alkalosis
C   lactic acidemia
D   warm extremities
E   hyperventilation

7.14   *Erysipelas*

A   is caused by staphylococcus
B   most commonly involves the shins
C   is gradual in onset
D   is usually diagnosed by isolation of organisms from the skin
E   responds to topical steroids

(Answers overleaf)

7.11 A **True**   however, cases in the over 65s account for 80 per cent
                    of deaths from *influenza*
     B **False**   there is no cross reactivity between strains and hence
                    the necessity for annual vaccination
     C **False**   serum *antibody* response begins in the second week
                    and peaks in the fourth week after initial vaccination
     D **False**   ageing of the immune system does not appear to
                    reduce efficacy of vaccination and it should be
                    recommended for sick and disabled old people if not
                    for all those over 65 years
     E **False**   annual immunisation is necessary
                                                       Brocklehurst, p. 96

7.12 A **True**   gram-negative anaerobic bacteria
     B **False**   gram-positive bacteria
     C **True**
     D **False**   Gram-positive bacteria
     E **True**   other gram-negative organisms which frequently
                    cause septicaemia are *Escherichia coli*, pseudomonas
                    and proteus
                                                       Harrison, p. 859

7.13 A **False**   low cardiac output and low central venous pressure
     B **False**   respiratory alkalosis and hyperventilation characterise
                    the early stages of shock. Perfusion failure in late
                    shock results in high grade lactic acidemia and
                    metabolic acidosis
     C **True**
     D **False**   extremities are cool and cyanotic
     E **False**   Hyperventilation characterises early stages
                                                       Harrison, p. 861

7.14 A **False**   *erysipelas* is an acute infection of the skin and
                    subcutaneous tissues caused by Group A *streptococci*
     B **False**   the commonest site of involvement is the face where
                    cutaneous infection originates from the upper
                    respiratory tract by way of small breaks in the skin
     C **False**   the onset is abrupt. The lesion spreads rapidly,
                    reaching its maximum extent in 3–6 days
     D **False**   the diagnosis is primarily clinical. Group A
                    streptococci may occasionally be isolated from the
                    respiratory tract or bloodstream
     E **False**   penicillin is the treatment of choice
                                                       Harrison, p. 932

7.15 Suppurative *parotitis* in the elderly

    A   is caused by streptococcus viridaus infection
    B   occurs with phenothiazines
    C   requires surgical intervention
    D   responds to penicillin
    E   occurs following general anaesthesia

7.16 *Pneumococcal pneumonia* may be associated with

    A   arthritis
    B   acute bacterial endocarditis
    C   encephalitis
    D   paralytic ileus
    E   impaired liver function

7.17 Chronic *osteomyelitis*

    A   may result in Brodie's abscess
    B   occurs after hip joint replacement
    C   is commonly due to gram-negative organisms
    D   is usually associated with penetrating wounds
    E   is optimally treated for 14 days with antimicrobials

(Answers overleaf)

7.15 A False   suppurative *parotitis* is generally associated with
              Staphylococcus aureus
     B True   occurs with any medications with atropine-like effect,
              i.e. phenothiazines and antihistamines
     C False   surgery is reserved for patients failing to respond to
              medical management, i.e. systemic antibiotics, gland
              massage and sialagogues
     D False   responds to systemic antimicrobial therapy with
              agents effective against *Staphylococcus Aureus*,
              i.e. penicillinase — resistant penicillin
     E True   occurs in elderly or chronically debilitated patients
              who have a dry mouth and decreased oral intake
              following general anaesthesia, surgery or
              medications (as above)
                                              Harrison, p 868

7.16 A True   in the elderly the joint may be swollen but not
              erythematous or painful. *Joint* swellings occurring in
              the presence of other sources of infection in an elderly
              person should always be aspirated
     B True   complicates *pneumococcal pneumonia* in fewer than
              0.5 per cent of cases
     C False   meningitis may occur
     D True   gaseous abdominal distention is commonly present
              and in severely ill patients may justify a diagnosis of
              paralytic ileus
     E True   impaired *liver* function tests occur in up to 25 per cent
              of patients with pneumococcal pneumonia,
              abnormal liver function tests are also associated with
              other infections in the elderly
                                       Kenny et al, Age and Ageing, 1984b
                                              Harrison, p. 920

7.17 A True   indolent infections of *bone* may remain localised for
              years within granulation tissue about a central
              necrotic area — *Brodie's abscess*
     B True   particularly in elderly patients and may occur many
              years after surgery
     C False   is most commonly due to *Staphylococcus aureus*
              infections
     D False   bone involvement follows haematogenous
              dissemination of infection
     E False   the optimal duration of treatment is not known but
              usually several months of antimicrobial therapy are
              necessary together with removal of devitalized bone
              and local drainage of abscess cavities
                                              Harrison, pp 925, 928

7.18 *Pneumonia* **due to Group A streptococci is characterised by**

    A   severe illness
    B   a preceding viral infection
    C   lobar consolidation
    D   serosanguinous empyema
    E   myalgia

7.19 *Escherichia Coli*

    A   is a gram-negative non-sporing rod
    B   is a normal commensal in the gastrointestinal tract
    C   accounts for over 75 per cent of urinary tract infections in the elderly
    D   is associated with metastatic infection in 30 per cent of bacteraemic patients
    E   is differentiated from other gram-negative bacteria on gram's stain

7.20 *Legionnaire's disease* **is characterised by**

    A   severe pneumonia
    B   positive sputum culture
    C   respiratory failure
    D   leucopenia
    E   unilateral pulmonary infiltrates

(Answers overleaf)

7.18 A **True**   patients are severely ill and often cyanosed
      B **True**   it usually occurs following a viral infection,
                     i.e. influenza
      C **False**   *bronchopneumonia*
      D **True**   characteristically thin, serosanguinous empyema fluid
                     accumulates early and rapidly
      E **True**

Harrison, p. 933

7.19 A **True**
      B **True**
      C **True**
      D **False**   5–10 per cent of *Escherichia coli* bacteraemic patients
                     develop metastatic manifestations in bone, brain, liver
                     and lung
      E **False**   culture and biochemical characterisation are
                     necessary

Harrison, p. 947

7.20 A **True**
      B **False**   routine bacteriological studies including blood and
                     sputum are negative and diagnosis depends on a four
                     fold or greater rise in serum *antibody* to a reciprocal
                     titre of at least 128
      C **True**
      D **False**   most patients have a modest granulocytosis and 20
                     per cent have leucocyte counts in excess of 20 000
                     per cubic millimetre
      E **True**   at initial presentation most patients have unilateral
                     parenchymal infiltrates which progress to involve
                     both *lungs* as the disease advances

Harrison, p. 985

8. Neurology

8.1 Causes of lethargy and stupor in *cerebral infarction* are

A presence of fever
B injudicious use of sedatives
C circulatory failure
D electrolyte imbalance
E fluid overload

8.2 The following are good predictors of return of motor function in the early stages of a completed *stroke*

A preservation of some voluntary movement
B slow return of function over the first few months
C flaccid paralysis persisting for the first 30 days
D substantial sensory loss
E brain stem infarct localised to the lateral medullary area

8.3 *Brain stem infarction* is associated with

A nausea and vomiting
B vertigo
C diplopia
D dysphagia
E ataxia

(Answers overleaf)

8.1 A **True**
    B **True**   injudicious use of sedatives, tranquillisers, narcotics
    C **True**
    D **True**
    E **True**   if this leads to *congestive cardiac failure* or
                  hyponatraemia

                                                          Cecil, p. 2063

8.2 A **True**
    B **False**   a slow return of function over weeks or months is
                  associated with less complete recovery
    C **False**   if flaccid paralysis persists from the onset with no
                  return of voluntary movement after 30–60 days, the
                  outlook for useful recovery is poor
    D **False**   substantial sensory loss implies poor recovery of
                  motor function and interferes with rehabilitation
    E **True**

                                                          Cecil, p. 2063

8.3 A **True**
    B **True**
    C **True**
    D **True**
    E **True**

                                                          Cecil, p. 2063

8.4   In surgery for cerebral atherothrombotic disease

A   carotid endarterectomy has become common practice for patients with symptoms appropriate to a stenosed atheromatous lesion in the lower cervical portion of the internal carotid artery

B   if the mortality and morbidity combination of cerebral angiography and carotid endarterectomy in a given centre exceeds 3 per cent, the patient will fare as well by medical management

C   a carotid endarterectomy at the level of the carotid sinus is of value even if there is an intracranial stenotic lesion equal in size to the neck stenosis

D   patients with vertebro-basilar symptoms do not benefit from surgery on simultaneously stenosed but asymptomatic carotid lesions

E   in the presence of a completed stroke immediate endarterectomy is indicated

8.5   A 72-year-old woman requires cholecystectomy. During the physical examination a right *carotid bruit* is detected, maximal in intensity near the angle of the jaw. With regard to the bruit, the most appropriate approach is

A   observation with no further studies

B   carotid arteriography

C   carotid endarterectomy

D   Doppler studies

E   cerebral vasodilator therapy

8.6   A *carotid bruit*

A   is an index of widespread arterial disease

B   is associated with an increased risk of stroke from the artery in which the bruit exists

C   is more common in females than in males

D   has an increased incidence with age

E   strongly indicates prophylactic endarterectomy as a prelude to open heart surgery

8.7   Which of the following statements concerning *cerebrovascular disease* is/are correct?

A   as life expectancy of the general population is increasing, so the incidence of stroke appears to be rising significantly

B   approximately one person in 6 will die as a consequence of cerebrovascular disease

C   atherosclerosis of the middle and the anterior cerebral arteries is the cause of most strokes

D   complete occlusion of the internal carotid artery usually produces a dense contralateral hemiparesis

E   chronic atrial fibrillation alone results in a five fold increased risk of stroke

(Answers overleaf)

8.4 A **True**
     B **True**
     C **False**   a *carotid endarterectomy* at the level of the carotid
                     sinus is of dubious advantage if there is evidence of a
                     stenotic or ulcerated lesion intracranially that equals
                     or exceeds in size that in the neck
     D **True**
     E **False**   carotid endarterectomy is not recommended in the
                     presence of a completed stroke or in the presence of
                     complete arterial occlusion

                                                        Cecil, p. 2064

8.5 A **True**   a neck bruit is an index of widespread arterial disease.
     B **False**   Stroke usually develops from arteries other than the
     C **False**   one in which the bruit exists. Patients with
     D **False**   asymptomatic bruits should be followed
     E **False**   conservatively

                                                        Cecil, p. 2064

8.6 A **True**
     B **False**   such bruits are associated with an increased risk of
                    stroke but the resultant stroke often develops in
                    arteries other than the one in which the bruit exists

     C **True**
     D **True**
     E **False**   cerebral ischaemic events after such major surgical
                    procedures are most often due to emboli initiated by
                    cardiopulmonary bypass rather than to hypertension
                    and haemodynamic focal ischaemia

                                                        Cecil, p. 2064

8.7 A **False**   the incidence of *stroke* has decreased probably due to
                    a decrease in deaths secondary to *hypertension* and
                    reduction in sequelae of *rheumatic fever*
     B **True**
     C **False**   the cause of most strokes is atherosclerosis of the
                    major extracranial arteries of the brain
     D **True**   but it may also be asymptomatic
     E **True**   there is a higher incidence with valvular heart disease
                                                        Cecil, p. 2050
                                                    Weksler, Stroke, 1983

8.8   The following cause concentric diminution *(tunnel vision)* of vision

    A   glaucoma
    B   senile macular degeneration
    C   papilloedema
    D   hysteria
    E   migraine

8.9   The following cause *central scotoma*

    A   senile macular degeneration
    B   optic atrophy due to vitamin B12 deficiency
    C   retinitis pigmentosa
    D   occipital pole lesions
    E   perisellar tumours

8.10   Clinical signs of Ramsey-Hunt syndrome (geniculate herpes zoster) include

    A   vesicles on the anterior fauces
    B   pain in the contralateral ear
    C   facial spasm
    D   hyperacusis
    E   ipsilater 12th nerve palsy

8.11   *Cataract* may be associated with

    A   senility
    B   glaucoma
    C   ophthalmitis
    D   trauma
    E   optic atrophy

8.12   Causes of *sudden blindness* are

    A   acute glaucoma
    B   retinal vein thrombosis
    C   myaesthenia gravis
    D   cranial arteritis
    E   retinal artery embolism

8.13   Causes of *paraplegia* in elderly patients include

    A   spinal artery occlusion
    B   sub-acute combined cord degeneration
    C   Paget's disease
    D   Guillain-Barré syndrome
    E   diabetes mellitus

(Answers overleaf)

8.8   A **True**
      B **False**   *central scotoma*
      C **True**
      D **True**
      E **True**

Burton, p. 101

8.9   A **True**   any retinal disease involving the macula
      B **True**
      C **False**   causes *tunnel vision*
      D **True**
      E **False**   cause *bitemporal hemianopia*

Burton, p. 101

8.10 A **True**   and auricle
      B **False**   ipsilateral ear and mastoid region
      C **True**   facial paresis and spasm
      D **True**   secondary paralysis of the nerve to the stapedius
                     muscle
      E **False**   ipsilateral taste loss in anterior two-thirds of tongue
                     due to involvement of chorda tympani and lingual
                     nerve

Cecil, pp 1656–1658

8.11 A **True**
      B **True**
      C **True**
      D **True**
      E **False**

Brocklehurst, pp 480–481

8.12 A **True**   other causes of *sudden blindness* in the elderly are
      B **True**   trauma, vitreous haemorrhage, retinal detachment,
      C **False**   cerebral infarction or haemorrhage and hypertensive
      D **True**   encephalopathy and hysteria
      E **True**

Burton, p. 105

8.13 A **True**
      B **True**
      C **True**   also vertebral collapse, disc prolapse, primary or
                     secondary neoplasm and vertebral tuberculous or
                     pyogenic infections
      D **True**
      E **False**

Cecil, pp 2142–2143

8.14   **Wasting of the small muscles of the right hand in an 80-year-old male is most commonly due to**

A   arthritis of the hand or wrist
B   cervical spondylosis
C   meningo-vascular syphilis
D   multiple sclerosis
E   syringomyelia

8.15   **Which of the following statements concerning the management of *chronic pain* is/are true**

A   early prompt treatment is the most effective means of controlling pain
B   minor analgesics are rarely beneficial and should be avoided
C   tolerance develops to all narcotic analgesics
D   drug combinations should be avoided
E   antidepressants should be reserved for patients with concomitant depression

8.16   **Which of the following statements regarding chronic *subdural haematoma* is/are true?**

A   neurological signs are always present at presentation
B   headache and lethargy are common presenting symptoms
C   the syndrome is common in chronic alcoholics
D   a negative CT scan excludes the diagnosis
E   they are a common cause of death in elderly patients

8.17   **Which of the following statements regarding *subdural haematoma* are true**

A   because of the reduction in the subarachnoid space with age, haematoma produces symptoms earlier in older patients
B   within 2–3 weeks the haematoma becomes encased in a highly vascular membrane
C   the walls of the haematoma may calcify
D   spontaneous reabsorption frequently occurs
E   anticoagulant therapy does not enhance the liability to bleed following trivial blows to the head

8.18   **If the *Wechsler Adult Intelligence Scale (WAIS)* indicates that an elderly patient has a markedly better verbal than performance IQ, possible explanations include which of the following**

A   Alzheimer's disease
B   multi-infarct dementia
C   depression
D   poor education
E   acute confusional state

(Answers overleaf)

8.14 A **True**
      B **True**
      C **False**   can cause it; but uncommon
      D **False**
      E **False**   does cause wasting of the small muscles of the hand
                      but not frequently in the elderly
                                          Brocklehurst, pp 285, 799

8.15 A **True**
      B **False**
      C **True**
      D **False**   drug combination treatment is often more effective
                      than single drug therapy but should be used
                      cautiously in elderly patients
      E **False**   the effects of minor analgesics and antidepressants
                      are additive
                                          Cecil, p. 143

8.16 A **False**
      B **True**
      C **True**
      D **False**   if the diagnosis is strongly suspected a radionuclide
                      brain scan or cerebral arteriography may be more
                      definitive
      E **False**
                                          Brocklehurst, pp 397–398

8.17 A **False**   the subarachnoid space tends to be larger in old age
                      and therefore haematoma may increase in size
                      considerably before producing obvious symptoms
      B **True**
      C **True**
      D **True**
      E **False**   disorders of haemostasis and anticoagulation both
                      enhance the liability to bleed following trauma
                                          Brocklehurst, pp 397–398

8.18 A **True**   in brain disease, performance disturbances appear
                      before verbal disturbances. Verbal tests measure
                      learning ability, while performance tests indicate the
                      capacity to meet new problems
      B **True**
      C **True**
      D **False**
      E **True**
                                          Cecil, p. 1980

8.19   *Creutzfeld-Jakob disease* is
  A   a slowly progressive disease
  B   frequently associated with ataxia, aphasia and visual
        disturbances
  C   accompanied by myoclonus
  D   the result of cortical degeneration caused by a
        transmissable agent
  E   characterised by 2 per second spike and wave activity

8.20   **The following are true of *lipofuscin***
  A   extracellular deposition of lipofuscin is part of general
        ageing in many tissues
  B   it is a yellow brown pigment
  C   it can be detected in glial cells in the first decade of life and
        thereafter increases in amount with age
  D   it can accumulate in large amounts during a variety of
        degenerative processes
  E   it is damaging to cells

8.21   *Pick's disease*
  A   results in dementia in middle and late life
  B   is characterised by diffuse cerebral atrophy
  C   is characterised pathologically by the accumulation of a
        globular argyrophilic mass close to the neuronal nucleus
  D   is clearly distinct from Alzheimer's disease on clinical
        grounds
  E   is less common than Alzheimer's disease

8.22   **The following are true of *Alzheimer's* senile dementia**
  A   the brain usually shows atrophy
  B   the brain usually weighs between 2000 and 2500 g
  C   atrophy is most marked in the parietal lobes
  D   argyrophilic plaques are rarely present
  E   neurofibrillary tangles and reactive gliosis are frequent
        findings

(Answers overleaf)

8.19 A **False** rapidly progressive, advancing day by day from its
            onset to a fatal termination, usually within a year
      B **True**   also paralysis of limbs
      C **True**   prominant myoclonic jerking of limbs and body occur
            at some stage of the disorder
      D **True**   of the late or slow virus variety
      E **False** is characterised by a distinctive mixture of slow and
            sharp waves on the EEG

                                                    Cecil, p. 192
                                            Brocklehurst, p. 315

8.20 A **False** intracellular deposition is part of general ageing in
            many tissues
      B **True**
      C **True**
      D **True**   it is known as 'wear and tear' pigment
      E **False** it is not harmful to cells but may be a pointer to the
            presence of potentially damaging aberrations of
            cellular material

                                            Brocklehurst, pp 269–270

8.21 A **True**
      B **False** severe atrophy is confined to frontal and temporal
            lobes
      C **True**   this distends the cell into a swollen ballooned form —
            the Pick cell
      D **False** is difficult to distinguish from Alzheimer's disease on
            clinical grounds
      E **True**

                                                    Cecil, p. 1982
                                            Brocklehurst, pp 278–279

8.22 A **True**
      B **False** 1000–1100 g
      C **False** frontal, temporal and occipital lobes
      D **False**
      E **True**   the important pathological changes are the
            appearance of argyrophilic *plaques* neurofibrillary
            tangles, neuronal loss and reactive *gliosis*

                                            Brocklehurst, pp 276–278
                                            Perry, Age Ageing, 1980

8.23 **Which of the following statements regarding *rigidity* in the elderly are true**

A   it occurs almost invariably in Parkinson's disease
B   it may be normally increased with age
C   rigidity and akinesia are a feature of phenothiazine-induced Parkinsonism
D   there is discontinuous activity in the involved muscles
E   it is associated with lesions of the subthalamic nucleus

8.24 ***Parkinson's disease* is characterised by which of the following?**

A   a deficiency of striatal dopamine
B   cholinergic hypoactivity in the basal ganglia
C   hypotonia
D   a tremor at rest which suppresses during sleep
E   postural instability

8.25 **Post-encephalitic *Parkinson's disease* is characterised by which of the following?**

A   neurofibrillary tangles in the basal ganglia
B   scarring in the floor of the fourth ventricle
C   antibodies to reovirus
D   CSF antibodies to measles virus
E   oculogyric crisis

8.26 ***Progressive supranuclear palsy* is characterised by the following**

A   rigidity and akinesia
B   tremor
C   external ophthalmoplegia
D   nuchal dystonia
E   limited eye movements during doll's eye test

8.27 **Which of the following statements regarding herpes zoster (shingles) is/are true?**

A   it is due to varicella virus
B   it is associated with activation of varicella virus latent in sensory ganglia
C   its increased incidence in the elderly may be associated with the decline in immunity in this age group
D   it frequently occurs in adults exposed to zoster
E   it frequently occurs in adults exposed to children with chicken pox

(Answers overleaf)

8.23 A **True**   rigidity is almost invariably present in the elderly with Parkinson's syndrome but may require careful attention to detail to elicit
    B **True**   the normal increase that may occur with age is readily distinguished by its uniformity at all joints
    C **True**
    D **False**   electromyography shows continued muscle activity
    E **False**   lesions of the subthalamic nucleus produce ballismus

Brocklehurst, pp 392–396

8.24 A **True**   the substantia nigra degenerates
    B **False**   dopamine deficiency allows for cholinergic hyperactivity in Parkinsonism. These patients respond to anticholinergic agents
    C **False**   rigidity and increased muscle tone
    D **True**
    E **True**   patients often exhibit difficulties in positioning themselves

Cecil, pp 2025–2026
Brocklehurst, pp 394–396

8.25 A **True**   tangles are found in the substantia nigra and locus caeruleus as well as the hypothalamus, reticular formation, lower brainstem and elsewhere
    B **True**   scarring in cerebral cortex, basal ganglia and in nuclei in the floor of the fourth ventricle
    C **False**
    D **False**   no virus has been identified in these patients
    E **True**

Brocklehurst, pp 394–396

8.26 A **True**
    B **False**   it resembles Parkinson's disease but tremor is rare
    C **True**   the presence of ophthalmoplegia is required for the diagnosis
    D **True**   especially neck hyperextension
    E **False**   a full range of eye movements are detected by the doll's eye test indicating that ophthalmoplegia is not due to a lesion of oculomotor nuclei or nerves

Cecil, p. 2027
Brocklehurst, pp 415–416

8.27 A **True**
    B **True**   the precise pathogenesis is unknown but this is the most likely hypothesis
    C **True**
    D **False**   it can occur but rarely
    E **False**   it can occur but rarely

Cecil, pp 2091–2093
Brocklehurst, pp 404–406
Faizallah, British Medical Journal, 1982

8.28   *Pagets* disease may be associated with

    A   headache
    B   intermittent tinnitus and vertigo
    C   urinary incontinence
    D   paraplegia
    E   sensorineural hearing loss

8.29   *Temporal arteritis* (giant cell arteritis)

    A   is the only arteritis with a predilection for the aged
    B   affects medium-sized vessels only
    C   is characterised histologically by granulomatous tissue containing epithelioid and multinucleate giant cells
    D   never involves the venous system
    E   is associated with underlying malignancy in 30 per cent of cases

8.30   Which of the following are true of vascular disease of the *spinal cord*

    A   elderly subjects are more commonly affected
    B   the commonest cause is occlusion of the posterior spinal artery
    C   the commonest signs are a mixture of sensory and upper and lower motor neurone defects
    D   dissecting aneurysm is the commonest cause of vascular damage
    E   anterior spinal artery occlusion results in a sharply defined area of infarction in the anterior two-thirds of the cord

8.31   Age-related changes result in

    A   a decline in olfactory function
    B   gross visual field changes
    C   impaired conjugate upward gaze
    D   altered doll's eye movement
    E   altered pupillary reactions to light

(Answers overleaf)

8.28 A **True**   probably due to increased blood flow through the external carotid artery
      B **True**
      C **True**   due to spinal cord compression
      D **True**   due to spinal cord compression
      E **True**   although eighth cranial nerve hearing loss has been attributed to compression of the eighth cranial nerve as the nerve traverses the canal in the temporal zone, this explanation appears unlikely since the facial nerve which parallels the course of the eighth nerve is rarely affected

                                                                Cecil, p. 1346
                                                       Brocklehurst, pp 772–773

8.29 A **True**
      B **False**   large arteries and small arterioles
      C **True**   plus chronic inflammatory cell infiltration and, in the acute stage, polymorphonuclear infiltration
      D **False**
      E **False**

                                                       Brocklehurst, pp 413–414

8.30 A **True**   but disorders of this type are uncommon at any age
      B **False**   anterior spinal artery
      C **True**
      D **False**   atheroma is the commonest cause but dissecting aneurysm, coarctation of the aorta, postoperative hypotension, emboli and spondylosis may all jeopardize the spinal cord circulation
      E **True**

                                                       Brocklehurst, pp 406–407

8.31 A **True**   there is good evidence of a substantial age related decline in *olfactory sensation*
      B **False**   no change in *visual fields*
      C **True**   *conjugate upward gaze* is often impaired and convergence limited in the elderly. Abnormal upward gaze is found in 30 per cent of neurologically normal old people and twice as many elderly patients with dementia
      D **False**   the *doll's head manoeuvre* is unaltered in the elderly
      E **False**   pupillary reactions to light are preserved though the *pupils* are usually smaller than in the young and may be slightly eccentric and irregular

                                                            Caird, pp 45–46

8.32 The following are present with increased frequency in normal ageing

A   jaw jerk
B   palmomental reflex
C   glabellar tap
D   extensor plantar responses
E   absent abdominal reflexes

8.33 The following is/are true of *cerebral blood flow* (CBF) in *dementia*

A   it is unchanged
B   psychological tests correlate poorly with CBF
C   it is reduced in the presence of cerebral atherosclerosis
D   it is of value in differentiating multi infarct from Alzheimer's type dementia
E   reduced CBF is more marked in frontal and temporal areas than in the rest of the cortex

8.34 The following is/are likely in a patient presenting with a slightly *painful red eye*

A   acute glaucoma
B   conjunctivitis
C   subconjunctival haemorrhage
D   acute iritis
E   episcleritis

8.35 Age change(s) in the *EEG* is/are

A   a decline in basic alpha rhythms
B   theta and delta slow wave activity in the left temporal area
C   generalised fast rhythms
D   generalised slow rhythms
E   3 per second spike and wave activity

8.36 The following is/are true of the confused elderly patient

A   most episodes of delirium are due to infections or cardiac failure
B   most elderly patients with acute confusion will recover
C   parietal and frontal lobe disorders may simulate a confusional state
D   depression may simulate a confusional state
E   detailed neurological investigation in the absence of neurological signs is indicated

(Answers overleaf)

8.32　A　**False**
　　　B　**True**
　　　C　**True**　　not specific to *Parkinsonism*; it is present in one-third of neurologically normal old people
　　　D　**False**　　the plantar responses are extensor only in the same circumstances as in the young
　　　E　**True**　　abdominal reflexes are more often absent than present

Caird, pp 47–48

8.33　A　**False**　　there is a significant reduction in CBF in patients with organic dementia
　　　B　**False**　　high correlation between psychological test scores and CBF
　　　C　**True**
　　　D　**False**　　some authors have reported a greater reduction in CBF for a given degree of dementia in *multi-infarct* than in *Azheimer's* cases whereas others were not able to confirm this
　　　E　**True**

Caird, p. 28
Kenny, Journal of Clinical and
Experimental Genontology, 1984

8.34　A　**False**　　presents with very *painful red eye*
　　　B　**True**
　　　C　**True**
　　　D　**False**
　　　E　**True**

Price, p. 1443

8.35　A　**True**　　though the dominant frequency does not fall below 8 Hz, the lower limit of normal
　　　B　**True**　　many normal elderly subjects show episodic, irregular slow wave activity
　　　C　**False**　　these indicate drug effects
　　　D　**False**　　these indicate a metabolic disorder
　　　E　**False**　　this indicates partial *epilepsy* (petit mal)

Caird, pp 58–59

8.36　A　**True**
　　　B　**True**
　　　C　**True**
　　　D　**True**
　　　E　**False**　　in the absence of focal neurological signs detailed investigation for an intracranial lesion gains little although the EEG may be helpful

Caird, pp 63–65

8.37   The following is/are true of bowel function after stroke

    A   *constipation* is frequently found
    B   faecal incontinence is rare
    C   if initially incontinent, patients rarely regain continence
    D   faecal incontinence is an important prognostic symptom
    E   constipation after stroke is drug induced

8.38   A predominantly *sensory neuropathy* occurs in

    A   vitamin B12 deficiency
    B   Guillain-Barré syndrome
    C   diabetes
    D   thiamine deficiency
    E   porphyria

8.39   A predominantly *motor neuropathy* occurs in

    A   diphtheria
    B   malignancy
    C   amyloid
    D   uraemia
    E   Charcot-Marie-Tooth syndrome

8.40   Papilloedema

    A   is a well documented feature of Guillain-Barré syndrome
    B   usually causes little disturbance of visual activity
    C   is an early feature of space occupying lesions of the cerebral
        hemispheres
    D   may be unilateral in malignant hypertension
    E   is a contraindication to lumbar puncture in a patient with
        normal pressure hydrocephalus

8.41   In chronic simple *glaucoma*

    A   loss of the nasal visual field is an early finding
    B   there is horizontal elongation of the physiological cup
    C   the most common presentation is a painful red eye
    D   pilocarpine is contraindicated
    E   peripheral iridectomy is seldom indicated

(Answers overleaf)

8.37 A **True**
      B **False**   *faecal incontinence* is present in up to a quarter of acute *stroke* patients
      C **False**   in over 80 per cent continence returns
      D **True**   poor prognostic symptom if present for more than 4 weeks
      E **False**   *constipation* after stroke is a combination of immobility, and hence slowing of food transit time, poor fluid intake, poor roughage intake and physical difficulties with toiletting

Caird, p. 92

8.38 A **True**
      B **False**   predominantly motor
      C **True**
      D **True**
      E **False**

Caird, p. 171
Impallomeni, Lancet, 1984

8.39 A **True**
      B **False**   predominantly sensory
      C **False**   predominantly sensory
      D **False**   predominantly sensory
      E **True**

Caird, p. 171

8.40 A **True**   may be due to reduced drainage of CSF associated either with impaired absorption or increased production of CSF
      B **True**
      C **False**   it occurs early in posterior fossa space occupying lesions
      D **True**
      E **False**   *lumbar puncture* is frequently used in the management of these patients

Cecil, pp 2300, 2309

8.41 A **True**
      B **False**   vertical elongation of the *physiological cup*
      C **False**   commonly presents with visual loss because it slowly 'eats' into peripheral visual fields
      D **False**   pilocarpine is used to constrict the *pupil* and increase the angle of the iris and anterior chamber and acetazolamide is used to reduce pressure
      E **False**   peripheral *iridectomy* produces a permanent channel between the iris and the anterior chamber

Brocklehurst, pp 476–478
Price, British Medical Journal, 1983

8.42   Factors indicating high risk subgroups for the development of *glaucoma* are

- A   diabetes mellitus
- B   a family history of glaucoma
- C   the presence of coronary artery disease
- D   central scotoma
- E   hypercalcaemia

8.43   The following is/are true of *herpes zoster ophthalmicus*

- A   ocular complications occur in less than 25 per cent of patients
- B   corneal perforation may occur up to 2 years after infection
- C   glaucoma is a complication
- D   spontaneous corneal perforation is a frequent complication
- E   topical antibiotics are contraindicated in management

8.44   In *giant cell arteritis*

- A   visual impairment is usually of abrupt onset
- B   the posterior ciliary arteries are frequently involved
- C   all patients with ischaemic optic neuritis should be assumed to have giant cell arteritis until otherwise proven
- D   the cherry red spot at the macule is frequently seen in opthalmic artery involvement
- E   blindness is usually preceded by symptoms of the disease

8.45   Which of the following statements is/are true

- A   3rd nerve palsy frequently accompanies a posterior communicating artery aneurysm
- B   in brain stem lesions, facial palsy frequently accompanies 6th nerve lesions
- C   the 6th nerve has a long intracranial course
- D   the pupil is usually fixed and dilated in a cavernous sinus lesion
- E   giant cell arteritis can cause isolated ocular nerve lesions

(Answers overleaf)

8.42 A **True**
     B **True**
     C **True**
     D **False**   peripheral field loss
     E **False**

The development of *glaucoma* is also associated with a history of bleeding requiring transfusion, age over 40 years and high myopia

Brocklehurst, pp 476–478
Price, British Medical Journal, 1983

8.43 A **False**   ocular complications occur in half of the patients
     B **True**
     C **True**   *glaucoma*, recurrent *uveitis*, corneal perforation, loss of corneal sensation, *keratitis* and corneal scarring are all complications
     D **False**   rare complication
     E **False**   the correct management involves use of topical steroids, antibiotics, anti-glaucoma therapy, artificial tears and in some instances, tarsorrhaphy

Brocklehurst, pp 405–406

8.44 A **True**
     B **True**
     C **True**
     D **False**   although the posterior ciliary arteries are frequently involved, the central retinal artery is much less commonly involved; once it enters the substance of the optic nerve, there is very little elastic tissue in its walls
     E **True**   but it may be the initial presenting sign

Cecil, pp 1871–1872

8.45 A **True**
     B **True**   in the brain stem, the 6th nerve fibres pass close to the nerve 7th nerve nucleus
     C **True**
     D **False**   When the 3rd nerve is involved in *cavernous sinus* lesions, the pupil is usually normal in size because both sympathetic and parasympathetic fibres are involved
     E **True**   *diabetes, hypertension, syphilis, giant cell arteritis* and blood dycrasias all cause intrinsic nerve lesions

Cecil, pp 2153–2154

8.46   Dystonic movements are associated with

A   rheumatic fever
B   Levodopa
C   renal failure
D   cerebral neoplasm
E   neuroleptic withdrawal

8.47   In elderly patients with _cerebral tumour_

A   papilloedema is a late sign
B   epileptic seizures are generalised
C   early morning headache is an early symptom
D   metastases from primary extracranial tumours are the commonest tumours
E   dexamethasone is contraindicated

8.48   _Communicating hydrocephalus_ is characterised by

A   urinary incontinence presenting late in the disease
B   a long history of dementia
C   dilated ventricles and cortical sulci
D   raised CSF fluid pressure at lumbar puncture
E   aqueduct stenosis

8.49   The following is/are true of eye signs in _brain stem death_

A   mydriasis is always a feature
B   the pupils show no response to bright light
C   bright light is needed when testing and the room should be darkened
D   testing corneal reflexes requires very firm pressure in suspected cases
E   pre-existing ocular disease may account for pupils failing to respond to light in suspected cases

8.50   In _subdural haematoma_ in elderly patients

A   the CSF is clear with an elevated protein content
B   the sub acute form most commonly occurs
C   the chronic form may be bilateral
D   a history of head injury is frequently obtained
E   headache rarely occurs

(Answers overleaf)

8.46 A **True**
      B **True**
      C **True** dystonic movements are associated with central nervous system complications of systemic metabolic disorders, i.e. hepatic or renal failure, hyperthyroidism
      D **True**
      E **True**

Brocklehurst, pp 281–284

8.47 A **True**
      B **False** focal seizures are most common
      C **False** headache is an uncommon symptom in elderly patients
      D **True** metastases, glioma and meningioma
      E **False** frequently used for symptomatic relief to reduce tumour size

Caird, pp 231–234

8.48 A **False** incontinence occurs early and out of proportion to the degree of *dementia*
      B **False** a short history of dementia
      C **False** increased ventricular size with normal or small sulci
      D **False** normal CSF pressure
      E **False** aqueduct stenosis occurs in non-communicating hydrocephalus

Editorial, Lancet, 1977

8.49 A **False** Mydriasis is not a feature of brain death — as can readily be ascertained in any morgue
      B **True** the important point is that they should show no response to light — a really bright light is needed so the room should be darkened
      C **True**
      D **True** a sterile throat swab is more suitable than a wisp of cotton
      E **True**

Pallis, British Medical Journal, 1983

8.50 A **False** commonly xanthochromia with an elevated protein content
      B **False** the chronic form most commonly occurs; the acute and subacute forms are uncommon in the elderly
      C **True**
      D **False** unusual to get a history of *head injury* in the elderly
      E **False** headache commonly occurs but less commonly in elderly than in young patients

Brocklehurst, pp 397–398

8.51 The following is/are true

A the ventral thalamic nucleus links fibres from the cerebellum and basal ganglia to the motor cortex

B ventral thalamic lesions enhance the tremor of Parkinson's disease

C internal capsular lesions affect both corticospinal and extrapyramidal systems

D vascular lesions of the substantia nigra result in hemiballismus

E the main influence of the basal ganglia on movement is directly through projections on the spinal cord

8.52 The anatomic components of the *basal ganglia* include

A caudate nucleus

B subthalamic nucleus

C motor cortex

D internal capsule

E putamen

8.53 *Spasticity*

A is most marked in antigravity muscles

B is due to hyperactivity of gamma motor neurons

C is not abolished by procaine injection

D is characterised by continous motor unit activity

E persists in relaxed muscle

(Answers overleaf)

8.51 A **True**   the ventrolateral and ventroanterior thalamic nuclei
form an essential link in the ascending fibre systems
from both the *basal ganglia* and the cerebellum to the
motor cortex

    B **False**   lesions in the ventral thalamus can both abolish the
tremor of *Parkinson's disease* and attenuate limb
dyskinesia or ataxia associated with cerebellar
disorders

    C **True**   the ascending thalamocortical fibres pass through the
internal capsule

    D **False**   vascular lesions of the subthalamic nucleus of Luys
result in *hemiballismus* in which the arm and leg of
the opposite side are thrown about in a violent fashion

    E **False**   the *basal ganglia* do not project directly to the spinal
cord but rather influence movement via the cerebral
cortex

Harrison, pp 92–93

8.52 A **True**   as an anatomic entity the basal ganglia have no
    B **True**   precise definition. However, together with the
    C **False**   recognised nuclear structures of the caudate nucleus,
    D **False**   they include putamen, globus pallidus, substantia
    E **True**   nigra and subthalamic nucleus of Luys, portions of the
red nucleus, superior colliculus (tectum), brainstem
reticular formation and amygdala

Harrison, p. 92

8.53 A **True**   leg extensors and arm flexors
    B **True**   it is due to hyperactivity of small gamma motor
neurones, resulting in increased sensitivity of the
spindle muscle fibres to stretch, but may be related in
some instances to excessive activity of the larger
alpha motor neurones

    C **False**   gamma spasticity is abolished by procaine, alpha
spasticity is not

    D **False**   rigidity is characterised by continuous motor unit
activity whereas spasticity is characterised by sudden
augmentation of tone with gradual yielding upon
quick movement and the absence of resistance upon
slow movement and on relaxed muscle

    E **False**

Harrison, p. 95

8.54 *Hypotonia* **is characteristically associated with**
   A   acute cerebellar lesions
   B   Guillain-Barré syndrome
   C   Parkinson's disease
   D   diffuse frontal lobe lesions
   E   hemiballismus

8.55 **Which of the following statements is/are true**
   A   *Lipofuscin* deposition in neuronal cells occurs only in
       severe dementia
   B   there is marked neuronal cell loss with ageing
   C   Lewy bodies are characteristically associated with
       idiopathic paralysis agitans
   D   neurofibrillary tangles are diagnostic of senile *dementia*
   E   senile plaques are common in patients less than 60 years
       old

8.56 *Shy-Drager syndrome* **is characteristically associated with**
   A   orthostatic hypotension
   B   urinary incontinence
   C   rigidity
   D   tremor
   E   atonic bladder

(Answers overleaf)

8.54 A **True**
     B **True**
     C **False**   *rigidity* is prominent in post encephalitic *Parkinson's* syndrome and paralysis agitans
     D **False**   rigidity occurs with diffuse cerebral disease, i.e. atherosclerotic or Alzheimer's senile dementia (Gegenhalten)
     E **True**   *hypotonia* occurs with lesions of the *basal ganglia*— particularly in association with choreiform movements

Harrison, p. 95

8.55 A **False**   a general phenomenon of ageing in many tissues is the intracellular deposition of granules of lipofuscin— a yellow brown autofluorescent pigment closely related to ceroid
     B **False**   there are many conflicting reports about whether neurones are lost from the brain. Marked neuronal cell loss does not occur but loss of smaller numbers of cells is difficult to ascertain because of likely cohort differences
     C **True**   *Lewy bodies* are normal inclusions in melanin-containing neurones principally in the mid brain and brain stem and are particularly associated with idiopathic paralysis agitans
     D **False**   they occur in normal ageing, Alzheimer's pre-senile and senile dementia
     E **False**   senile *plaques* and *neurofibrillary* tangles are uncommon in patients less than 60 years old

Brocklehurst, pp 269, 271–275

8.56 A **True**   *Shy-Drager syndrome* is an uncommon clinical
     B **True**   syndrome consisting of mild extrapyramidal
     C **True**   movement disorders, orthostatic hypotension, atonic
     D **True**   bladder, *incontinence* and other features of damage to
     E **True**   the autonomic nervous system. Pathologically some cases resemble olivopontocerebellar atrophy, and some resemble more diffuse system degeneration. In the majority there is loss of intermediolateral spinal neurones

Brocklehurst, pp 282–283

8.57 *Lateral medullary syndrome* **is characterised by**
A ischaemia in the territory of the posterior superior cerebellar artery
B contralateral limb ataxia
C Horner's syndrome
D facial pain and temperature loss
E contralateral trunkal pain and temperature loss

8.58 **In elderly patients atherosclerotic dementia is**
A the main cause of dementia
B rarely associated with Alzheimer's senile dementia
C characterised by reduced cortical choline acetyltransferase activity
D easily clinically differentiated form Alzheimer's dementia
E characterised by personality changes early in the disease

8.59 *Creutzfeldt-Jacob disease* **is characteristically associated with**
A a genetic predisposition
B onset between 50 and 60 years
C myoclonic jerking
D peripheral neuropathy
E weight loss

(Answers overleaf)

8.57 A **False**   *Wallenburg's syndrome (lateral medullary syndrome)* results from ischaemia in the territory of the posterior inferior cerebellar artery
      B **False**   ipsilateral limb ataxia
      C **True**   ipsilateral *Horner's syndrome*
      D **True**   ipsilateral facial pain and temperature loss due to involvement of the fifth cranial nerve nucleus
      E **True**   contralateral findings consist of impaired pain and temperature loss which spares from the face

Other features are vertigo and vomiting at the onset, paralysis of the larynx, pharynx and palate due to 10th nerve involvement, and nystagmus

Cecil, pp 2058, 2063–2064

8.58 A **False**   less than 20 per cent of cases are due to *atherosclerotic dementia*, 50 per cent or more to *Alzheimer's senile dementia* and 20 per cent or more to mixed forms and 10 per cent to other causes
      B **False**   particularly in older subjects the presence of both forms in the same patient (mixed) makes differentiation between atherosclerotic and Alzheimer's dementia difficult
      C **False**   reductions in cortical choline acetyl-transferase activity occur in specific association with Alzheimer's disease, but they are not found consistently in multi-infarct dementia
      D **False**
      E **False**   personality is retained in atherosclerotic dementia until relatively late in the disease compared with Alzheimer's where change in personality occurs much earlier

Kenny, Journal of Clinical
and Experimental Gerontology, 1984
Perry, Age and Ageing, 1980

8.59 A **True**   there are several reports of families with an autosomal dominant pattern of inheritance. In 10 per cent of one series at least one other family member was affected and this is probably the result of viral infection superimposed on a pre-existing genetically determined dysfunction or vulnerability
      B **True**   although it may occur in much older subjects
      C **True**
      D **False**
      E **True**

Initially symptoms such as fatigue, anxiety, apathy, irritability and confusion often occur. These are followed by severe dementia, *myoclonic jerking*, rigidity, motor tract damage and assymetric reflexes. Weight loss and sleep disturbance occur in 12 to 15 per cent of cases.

Brocklehurst, p. 315

8.60   In *normal pressure hydrocephalus*
- A   features result from anterior horn enlargement
- B   CSF pressure is invariably elevated
- C   frontal lobe cortical atrophy is marked
- D   absorption of CSF is decreased
- E   surgery is always indicated

8.61   Clinical features of *pseudodementia* include
- A   a long history of symptoms before initial consultation
- B   rapid progression of symptoms
- C   early loss of social skills
- D   patchy memory loss
- E   prior history of psychopathology

8.62   *Paratonia* in the elderly is
- A   rare
- B   most marked during passive movements
- C   responsible for reported frequency of areflexia
- D   characterised by constant rigidity
- E   reduced if movements are performed slowly

(Answers overleaf)

8.60 A **True**   enlarged anterior horns of the lateral ventricles
compress surrounding areas resulting in behavioural
changes typical of frontal lobe damage. Gait, reflex
and bladder changes are due to stretching of motor
fibres to the legs and autonomic fibres — both of
which run in close proximity to the anterior horns

   B **False**
   C **False**   the classical appearance is prominent ventricular
dilation in the absence of cortical atrophy
   D **True**   absorption of CSF is characteristically decreased in
normal pressure hydrocephalus, and a cisternogram
may demonstrate this defect. A radioactive albumin
tracer is injected via a spinal tap into the subarachnoid
space and the flow is followed by subsequent brain
scans — an abnormal cisternogram is where tracer
enters the ventricles within 6 hours but fails to
circulate out within 24 hours, remaining up to 48
hours
   E **False**   the best candidates for ventricular shunting show
substantial *gait* disturbance but minimal cognitive
change

                                   Editorial, Lancet, 1977

8.61 A **False**   duration of symptoms before consultation is long in
dementia but short in *pseudodementia*
   B **True**   the opposite is true of dementia
   C **True**
   D **True**   specific memory gaps are unusual in dementia
   E **True**

                              Brocklehurst, pp 319–320

8.62 A **False**   is commonly found in old age and is also known as
gegenhalten
   B **True**   it is characterised by excessive motor tone during
passive manipulation of the limbs and may be
accentuated by rapid passive flexion and extension
   C **True**
   D **True**   the *rigidity* of gegenhalten is constant in contrast with
the plastic type of rigidity in Parkinsonism
   E **True**

                                   Brocklehurst, p. 392
                                 Impallomeni, Lancet, 1984

8.63 **Late onset *epilepsy* in elderly subjects**

A   is most commonly associated with cerebral tumour
B   may mimic thalamic syndrome
C   is associated with post ictal paresis in 15 per cent
D   is frequently resistant to anticonvulsant monotherapy
E   is associated with prolonged confusion in 15 per cent

8.64 **Persistent pain during the early weeks after *amputation* is usually due to which of the following**

A   phantom limb
B   neuroma
C   causalgia
D   ischaemic stump
E   arterial emboli

8.65 **An elderly patient has *hearing* difficulty. Using Weber's test (vibrating tuning fork placed at the centre of the forehead), the sound is better heard in the left ear. Using Rinnes test bone conduction is greater than air conduction in the left ear. Which of the following is/are true**

A   sensorineural deafness is present bilaterally
B   right conductive nerve deafness is present
C   there may be wax in the left ear
D   a diminished right corneal reflex may be present
E   the patient may have nystagmus on conjugate deviation of the eyes to the left

(Answers overleaf)

8.63 A **False**   the commonest cause is cerebrovascular disease —
                   tumour is responsible for 28 per cent of cases over 60
                   and only 7 per cent of cases over 70 years
     B **True**   pain in a hemiplegic limb is usually due to *subluxation*
                   but may be a manifestation of either post infarction
                   sensory epilepsy or the thalamic *syndrome of
                   Dejerine and Roussy* — in both the latter cases the
                   pain occurs with minimal or no stimulus to the
                   affected side and is relieved by anticonvulsant
                   therapy; therefore distinguishing between the
                   disorders is often difficult
     C **True**   *post ictal paresis* (*Todd's palsy*) is much more
                   common in the elderly and may last up to 4 days
     D **False**   patients generally respond well to monotherapy
     E **True**   15 per cent have ictal or post ictal confusion lasting for
                   longer than 24 hours and up to 7 days

Kenny, Geriatric Medicine, 1982
Godfrey, Age and Ageing, 1982
Roberts, Age and Ageing, 1982

8.64 A **True**
     B **True**
     C **True**
     D **True**
     E **False**

Cecil, p. 318

8.65 A **False**   because the *Weber's test* localises sound to the left
                   ear this indicates that there is a right nerve deafness
                   or a left conductive *deafness*. *Rinnes test* indicates
                   that bone conduction is greater than air conduction on
                   the left and therefore a left sided conductive deafness
     B **False**
     C **True**   causing conductive deafness
     D **True**   this suggests an acoustic neuroma
     E **True**   if there is a tumour at the *cerebello-pontine angle*,
                   there may be nystagmus, but this is likely to be
                   present when looking to the side of the lesion (in this
                   case the right)

Cecil, p. 1959

8.66   The following is/are true of *senile macular degeneration*

    A   retinal pigment epithelium is destroyed

    B   retinal detachment occurs

    C   neovascularisation is rare

    D   visual recovery usually occurs

    E   laser photocoagulation is of most value if the fovea is involved.

8.67   Brachial neuralgia

    A   is the commonest cause of partial brachial plexus lesions in the elderly

    B   carries a poor prognosis

    C   is caused by viral infection

    D   is associated with transverse myelitis

    E   responds to steroid therapy

(Answers overleaf)

8.66 A **True**   blood vessels from the choroid grow between the
                    choroid and *retina* in the posterior pole of the eye
                    leading to destruction of the posterior retina
     B **True**
     C **False**   the cause of neovascularisation is unknown but it
                    appears to be the final stage of a series of events at
                    the level of *Bruck's membrane* (the transparent inner
                    layer of the choroid) which is thought to occur with
                    ageing. This consists of deposition of debris derived
                    from retinal pigment epithelium and basement
                    membrane reduplication of the pigment epithelium,
                    which in turn induces infiltration by macrophages
     D **False**   visual recovery is rare because of extensive
                    destruction of tissues
     E **False**   in most patients, the complex of new vessels lies
                    beneath the *fovea* and destruction of tissue in this site
                    leads to severe visual loss; only 5 to 10 per cent of
                    patients in whom the neovascular complex does not
                    underline the fovea will benefit from treatment
                              Bird, British Medical Journal, 1983

8.67 A **False**   *cervical spondylosis* is the commonest cause of
                    partial *brachial plexus* lesions in the elderly
     B **False**   brachial neuralgia carries a good prognosis — 80 per
                    cent recovery within 2 years and 90 per cent within 3
                    years of onset
     C **False**   the aetiology is unknown although the relationship to
                    viral infections affecting other systems is striking
     D **False**   brachial neuralgia is an acute multiple brachial
                    neuropathy resulting in upper, middle or lower plexus
                    lesions
     E **False**
                                              Cecil, p. 2156

8.68 *Diogenes syndrome* **is associated with**
- **A** manic-depressive episodes
- **B** visual hallucinations
- **C** alcoholism
- **D** bereavement
- **E** self neglect

8.69 **The following is/are true of chronic open angle** *glaucoma*
- **A** temporal visual field loss is an early feature
- **B** pathological 'cupping' rarely occurs
- **C** digital tonometry is a reliable bedside test
- **D** peripheral iridectomy is frequently indicated
- **E** blindness rarely occurs

(Answers overleaf)

8.68 A **False**   *Diogenes syndrome* does not fit easily into
      B **False**   conventional psychiatric classification. It occurs in the
      C **True**   elderly and has social more than medical implications.
      D **True**   It is characterised by social isolation and extreme self
      E **True**   neglect. There is a female preponderance, an
                       association with bereavement and higher socio-
                       economic class and no real answer to the problem! It
                       must be differentiated from the senile paranoid state,
                       occult alcoholism, a dementing process and
                       depression.

Kafetz, Journal of the American
Geriatric Society, 1983

8.69 A **False**   loss of the nasal field is an early finding
      B **False**   pathological cupping results from the gradual
                       increase in depth as the cribriform fascia is forced
                       posteriorly by the increased pressure
      C **False**   digital tonometry should be performed but it is
                       unreliable as it may appear normal despite raised
                       intraocular pressure
      D **True**
      E **False**   both chronic open angle or closed angle *glaucoma*
                       remain important causes of *blindness* in the elderly —
                       up to 20 per cent of new registrations

Brocklehurst, pp 476–479
Price, British Medical Journal, 1983

9. Renal disease

9.1 The following is/are true of *dipstick* urine testing
A a distinct colour change occurs at 50 mg protein per litre
B testing is more accurate with dilute urine
C 'dipsticks' respond best to light chain protein fragments
D late afternoon is the optimum testing time
E a colour change of the 3+ level occurs at 300 mg protein per litre

9.2 The following is/are true of *renal* disease
A bleeding from the renal pelvis produces isolated haematuria and significant proteinuria
B analgesic nephropathy produces isolated haematuria and modest proteinuria
C white blood cell casts are particularly common in pyelonephritis
D red blood cell casts indicate bleeding into the nephron
E hyaline casts occur in dehydration

9.3 The ratio of blood *urea* nitrogen (BUN) to *creatinine* is elevated in
A dehydration
B gastrointestinal blood loss
C adrenocortical steroid therapy
D impaired tubular function
E tetracycline administration

(Answers overleaf)

9.1 A **False**   *dipsticks* may register a trace result in response to 50 mg protein per litre, but a distinct colour change of 1+ occurs at 300 mg per litre

   B **False**   *proteinuria* may be missed if the urine is very dilute, therefore fasting morning samples, when urine is most concentrated, are best studied

   C **False**   dipsticks respond best to albumin; a negative result can occur when large amounts of other protein or protein fragments such as light chains, are excreted

   D **False**   early morning fasting samples are best
   E **False**

Harrison, pp 2311–212

9.2 A **False**   bleeding from the *renal* pelvis produces isolated *haematuria*, without significant proteinuria, cells or urinary casts

   B **True**
   C **True**   they also indicate *nephritis* associated with systemic lupus erythematosus and transplant rejection

   D **True**   red blood cells in the tubule lumen are trapped in a cylindrical mold of gelled protein and produce casts which are conclusive evidence of bleeding into the nephron

   E **True**   heavy albuminuria or dehydration can cause showers of transparent, refractile 'hyaline' casts

Harrison, pp 213–214

9.3 A **True**
   B **True**
   C **True**
   D **False**
   E **True**   normally, the ratio of blood urea nitrogen (BUN) to creatinine is 10:1; with depletion of extracellular fluid, and any of the above mentioned factors, the ratio is elevated

Harrison, p. 215

9.4   An elderly house bound widow was found on the floor with evidence of an extensive right sided hemiplegia and oliguria. The following implicate *dehydration* rather than *acute tubular necrosis* (ATN) as the cause of oliguria

A   urine osmolality less than 300 mosmol/kg
B   urine sodium 60 mmol/l
C   supine blood pressure of 100/60 mmHg
D   urea U/P ratio of 10
E   Serum urea exceeding serum creatinine by 12 fold

9.5   Short-term *dialysis* is indicated when

A   serum potassium exceeds 5 mmol/l
B   hypercalcaemia is uncontrolled
C   blood urea is slowly rising
D   arterial pH is less than 7.29
E   there is salicylate poisoning

9.6   The following cause *renal vein thrombosis*

A   renal amyloid
B   dehydration
C   nephrotic syndrome
D   myxoedema
E   hypernephroma

9.7   The following may cause *nephrotic syndrome* in the elderly

A   diabetes mellitus
B   bacterial endocarditis
C   myxoedema
D   extra-renal malignancy
E   constrictive pericarditis

9.8   A 73-year-old retired ward sister was investigated for weight loss and fatigue. Urinalysis revealed 10 white cells per ml, occasional red blood cells and *Escherichia coli* in concentrations less than 10^3 colonies per ml. The following may be responsible for the urinary findings

A   lower urinary tract infection
B   analgesic nephropathy
C   chronic pyelonephritis
D   renal calculi
E   diuretics

(Answers overleaf)

9.4 A **False**   *urine osmolality* exceeding 500 mosmo1/kg of water
                   is in keeping with dehydration. However, osmolality
                   of less than 350 mosmo1/kg suggests acute tubular
                   necrosis (ATN)

    B **False**   with reduction of glomerular flow rate and preserved
                   tubular function, the urinary sodium is less than 20
                   mmol/l — concentrations greater than 40 mmol/l
                   imply tubular damage

    C **False**   supine blood pressure of 100/60 is consistent with
                   either diagnosis

    D **True**   U/P (urine/plasma) ratio for urea is in excess of 8 and
                   less than 2 in pre-renal and acute tubular necrosis
                   respectively; whereas U/P ratio for creatinine exceeds
                   40 or is less than 20 respectively

    E **True**

                                              Harrison, pp 215–216

9.5 A **False**   *hyperkalaemia* exceeding 7 mmol/l
    B **True**
    C **False**   rapidly rising blood urea
    D **False**   arterial pH less than 7.15
    E **True**

It is difficult to make hard and fast rules about indications for
dialysis — a combination of factors may indicate the need for short
term *dialysis* where single factors would not

                                                  Harrison, p. 1619

9.6 A **True**
    B **True**
    C **True**   any cause of nephrotic syndrome
    D **True**
    E **True**

                                              Harrison, pp 1664–1665

9.7 A **True**   other causes of *nephrotic syndrome* in the elderly are
    B **True**   amyloidosis, lymphoma, dysproteinaemia,
    C **True**   *staphylococcal septicaemia*, renal artery stenosis,
    D **True**   renal vein thrombosis, renal carcinoma and inferior
    E **True**   vena caval thrombosis

                                                  Harrison, p. 1636

9.8 A **False**   the patient has a *'sterile pyuria'* — the concentration of
                   significant pathogens should be greater than 10^5
                   colonies per ml

    B **True**
    C **True**
    D **True**
    E **True**   diuretics, analgesics and iron sorbitol citric acid
                   complex (Jectofer) may all give rise to 'sterile pyuria'

                                                  Harrison, p. 1598

9.9   The following are causes of *small kidneys*

 A   chronic glomerulonephritis
 B   nephrotic syndrome
 C   acute pyelonephritis
 D   chronic pyelonephritis
 E   analgesic nephropathy

9.10   A 78-year-old retired school mistress presented with hypercalcaemia, plasma creatinine 129 mmol/l and *nephrocalcinosis*. Which of the following disorders might be responsible

 A   primary hyperparathyroidism
 B   renal neoplasm
 C   pulmonary tuberculosis
 D   sarcoidosis
 E   papillary necrosis

9.11   The following are characteristic of the evolution of the *nephrogram* in renal disease

 A   increasing density with time — renal obstruction
 B   faint persisting nephrogram — chronic pyelonephritis
 C   no nephrogram — acute tubular necrosis
 D   dense persisting nephrogram — renal infarction
 E   no nephrogram — anuric glomerulonephritis

9.12   Neurological complications of *renal failure* include

 A   dementia
 B   peripheral neuropathy
 C   myopathy
 D   cranial neuropathy
 E   epilepsy

9.13   The following are true of renal function with advancing age

 A   decreased *glomerular filtration rate*
 B   increased *renal plasma flow*
 C   narrowing of major renal vessels
 D   decreased tubular reabsorptive capacity
 E   increased tubular excreting capacity

(Answers overleaf)

9.9   A **True**
      B **False**   cause large kidenys
      C **False**   usually cause large kidneys
      D **True**
      E **True**   *Kidney size* diminishes with ageing; the mean length
                      in subjects over 80 years being 12.5 mm

Burton, p. 163

9.10 A **True**
      B **True**
      C **False**   *renal tuberculosis* can result in localised
                      nephrocalcinosis but does not give rise to
                      hypercalcaemia
      D **True**
      E **False**   again, this does not cause hypercalcaemia in the face
                      of normal plasma creatinine levels

Cecil, pp 570, 574

9.11 A **True**   also occurs with hypotension, ischaemia, and severe
                      glomerulonephritis
      B **True**
      C **False**   in *acute tubular necrosis* the nephrogram is
                      immediate, dense and persisting
      D **False**   *renal infarct* is usually associated with no nephrogram
      E **True**

Burton, p. 163

9.12 A **True**
      B **True**
      C **True**
      D **True**
      E **True**

Burton, p. 157

9.13 A **True**   this is due to either a decreased functional capacity of
                      the glomeruli, or decreased renal plasma flow
                      obstruction
      B **False**
      C **True**   narrowing of both major and minor renal vessels
                      reduces *glomerular filtration* rate
      D **True**
      E **False**   both tubular excretory and reabsorptive capacity
                      decreases with age

Brocklehurst, pp 609–610

9.14 *Chronic pyelonephritis* **in elderly subjects is**

A   the commonest cause of renal disease
B   present in up to 20 per cent of post-mortem cases
C   caused by haematogenous spread of infection
D   caused by ascending infection
E   rarely asymptomatic

9.15 *L-forms* **of bacteria**

A   have a solid wall structure
B   emerge from bacteria exposed to antibiotics
C   have a high virulence
D   multiply rapidly in common broths used for bacterial cultivation
E   are rarely isolated in elderly patients with chronic urinary infections

9.16 *Renal papillary necrosis* **is**

A   uncommon in the elderly
B   detected by macroscopic urine examination
C   associated with haematuria
D   associated with fever
E   characterised by a slowly progressive course

9.17 **The following cause** *papillary necrosis*

A   phenacetin abuse
B   renal tuberculosis
C   multiple myeloma
D   pelvic irradiation
E   obstructive uropathy

(Answers overleaf)

9.14 A **True**
     B **True**
     C **True**
     D **True**
     E **False**   it is frequently asymtomatic. *Pyelonephritis* is diagnosed clinically in one fifth of cases detected at autopsy. In many cases it is not possible to detect bacteria in the urine despite progressive renal infection

Brocklehurst, pp 612–614

9.15 A **False**   the *L-forms* are bacterial cells without a solid wall structure. Bacteria change into L-forms after exposure to agents which damage the cell surface, i.e. antimicrobial agents and enzymes
     B **True**
     C **False**   L-forms have a low virulence but after returning to their normal bacterial forms the virulence is restored
     D **False**   they require their own cultivation techniques during which they return to their 'normal' forms
     E **False**   L-forms have been isolated in most cases in old patients with chronic *urinary infections*, often with severe underlying diseases

Brocklehurst, p. 614

9.16 A **False**   *renal papillary necrosis* is not uncommon in the elderly. It can be defined as a severe form of *chronic pyelonephritis* with ischaemic necrosis of papillae and the medullary pyramid
     B **True**   necrotic papillae migrate through the urinary passages and are often detected macroscopically in the urine
     C **True**   patients suffer from *haematuria*, urinary colic and fever
     D **True**
     E **False**   the disease often has a rapid course resulting in *uraemia* and death

Brocklehurst, p. 617

9.17 A **True**   in an autopsy series of 111 cases of *papillary necrosis*, 52 per cent were related to *phenacetin* abuse
     B **True**
     C **True**   *dysproteinaemia*
     D **True**
     E **True**
25 per cent of cases are attributable to diabetes whilst other causes include vascular lesions, *acute pyelonephritis* and sickle cell disease

Brocklehurst, p. 617

9.18 The following *renal stones* are radio-opaque

    A   calcium
    B   uric acid
    C   xanthine
    D   matrix
    E   cystine

9.19 *Acute glomerulonephritis* in the elderly

    A   is uncommon
    B   is limited to streptococcal infection
    C   commonly causes death due to circulatory congestion
    D   is commonly associated with hypertension
    E   is rarely accompanied by proteinuria

9.20 The following have an inhibitory effect on the sacral micturition reflex

    A   frontal lobe
    B   posterior hypothalamus
    C   midbrain
    D   anterior pons
    E   pelvic parasympathetic nerves

(Answers overleaf)

9.18 A **True**
     B **False**
     C **False**
     D **False**
     E **True**
Magnesium-ammonium phosphate and silicate stones are also
radio-opaque

Burton, pp 161–162

9.19 A **True**   although recent reports indicate that it is much more
                    common than generally realised
     B **False**   the aetiology of the disease in older patients is diverse
                    and not limited to *streptococcal infection* and the
                    prognosis is not as unfavourable as was generally
                    believed
     C **True**   the commonest cause of death is *pulmonary oedema*
                    secondary to circulatory congestion. Since many old
                    people have a variety of concomitant degenerative
                    diseases such as diabetes, congestive heart failure,
                    hypertension and peripheral vascular disease, the
                    tendency is to attribute markers of
                    glomerulonephritis, such as the presence of
                    haematuria, proteinuria, red blood cell casts and
                    azotemia to the aforementioned. Hence many cases of
                    acute pyelonephritis are not diagnosed ante-mortem
     D **False**
     E **False**

Brocklehurst, p. 617

9.20 A **True**
     B **False**   facilitatory effect
     C **True**
     D **False**   facilitatory effect
     E **False**   the parasympathetic nerves carry afferent fibres of the
                    sacral *micturition reflex* to the second, third and
                    fourth sacral segments of the spinal cord which is
                    either inhibited or facilitated by the ascending series
                    of centres mentioned

Brocklehurst, pp 628–629

9.21   The following is/are characteristic of the *neurogenic bladder*

    A   cauda equina lesions are associated with an uninhibited bladder

    B   frontal lobe lesions are associated with an autonomic bladder

    C   diabetes mellitus is associated with a reflex bladder

    D   spinal cord lesions are associated with an autonomous bladder

    E   tabes dorsalis is associated with an autonomous bladder

9.22   An *unstable bladder* is associated with

    A   prostatic enlargement

    B   diabetes mellitus

    C   vaginal repair operation

    D   reflex neurogenic bladder

    E   cauda equina lesions

9.23   *Micturating cystourethrography* demonstrates

    A   causes of stress incontinence

    B   neurogenic and non neurogenic causes of incontinence

    C   spastic bladder outlet

    D   urethral stricture

    E   reflex incontinence

(Answers overleaf)

9.21 A **False**   *cauda equina* lesions are associated with an
                    autonomous bladder—where both afferent and
                    efferent sides of parasympathetic innervation are
                    destroyed. The bladder empties inconsistently and
                    inefficiently from time to time as a result of local and
                    axonal reflexes

     B **False**   frontal lobe lesions are associated with an *uninhibited
                    bladder*—sensation is retained but the ability to
                    inhibit spontaneous contractions is lost. This is a
                    common cause of incontinence in the very old

     C **False**   *diabetes mellitus* and *tabes dorsalis* are both
                    associated with an *atonic bladder* caused by
                    destruction of posterior nerve roots — some power
                    and voluntary micturition remain but the patient is
                    unaware of bladder filling and hence the bladder
                    becomes overdistended leading to retention and
                    overflow

     D **False**   complete spinal cord lesions are associated with a
                    reflex bladder—sacral reflex is intact but influences of
                    higher centres are abolished and the bladder empties
                    incontinently from time to time

     E **False**

                                                    Brocklehurst, pp 629–630

9.22 A **True**   an *unstable bladder* develops instrinsic contractions
     B **False**   in response to stimuli such as movement, coughing,
     C **True**   and filling with cold water
     D **True**
     E **False**

                                                    Brocklehurst, p. 630

9.23 A **True**   genuine *stress incontinence* with abnormal descent of
                    the bladder base on assuming the erect position and
                    wide funnelling of the bladder outlet during
                    micturition is usually well demonstrated

     B **True**

     C **True**   this is shown as shelving — such as is associated with
                    spasticity of the striated muscles of the pelvic
                    diaphragm

     D **True**   this will be apparent, as with all causes of *bladder
                    outlet obstruction*, by the presence of trabeculation,
                    cellule, and diverticulae formation together with the
                    radiographic demonstration of urethral stricture

     E **True**   functional causes of obstruction such as reflex and
                    uninhibited neurogenic *bladders* demonstrate the
                    above findings

                                                    Brocklehurst, pp 633–635

9.24   *Senile vaginitis*

A   is best treated with oral oestrogen and progesterone medication

B   is rarely associated with urethritis

C   always results in urinary incontinence

D   is best treated by pelvic floor exercises

E   is always associated with trigonitis

9.25   **Poor *bladder function* and leakage is**

A   only found in association with neurogenic bladder disorders

B   always accompanied by incontinence

C   related to increasing frequency of nocturia with age

D   associated with immobility

E   uncommon after 65 years

9.26   *Atrophic vaginitis* **often presents with**

A   pruritis

B   blood-stained vaginal discharge

C   dysuria

D   urinary urgency

E   frank vaginal bleeding

9.27   *Carcinoma of the cervix* **is**

A   most frequent in the fourth decade

B   an adenocarcinoma in 90 per cent of cases

C   significantly related to late onset coitus

D   the commonest genital cancer

E   commoner in lower socio-economic groups

(Answers overleaf)

9.24 A **False**   where possible locally applied *oestrogen creams* are preferable
      B **False**   is frequently associated with urethritis and trigonitis — which may reflect the common embryological origin of the tissues
      C **False**   but there is a strong association between incontinence and senile vaginitis
      D **False**
      E **False**

Brocklehurst, pp 662–664

9.25 A **False**   in one study, over 40 per cent of elderly women, without evidence of neurological dysfunction, had leak and/or *bladder dysfunction* — it appears that a poorly functioning bladder is a common accompaniment of old age even among those not suffering from incontinence
      B **False**
      C **True**   *nocturnal frequency* increases with age and is twice as common in patients over 65 years as under. In younger subjects nocturia closely correlates with the presence of infection — this is not the case in older subjects
      D **True**   *incontinence* in particular is associated with *immobility* — over 80 per cent of incontinent elderly patients are non-ambulant
      E **False**

Brocklehurst, pp 635–636

9.26 A **True**
      B **True**
      C **True**   and *urinary frequency*
      D **True**
      E **False**   frank vaginal bleeding is usually due to another cause and even bloodstained *vaginal discharge* should not be assumed to be secondary to vaginitis until other causes of post menopausal bleeding have been excluded

Brocklehurst, pp 662–664

9.27 A **False**   occurs most frequently in the sixth decade
      B **False**   *squamous carcinoma* accounts for 95 per cent of primary neoplasms
      C **False**   coitus and an early age of onset of coitus are major prerequisites for the disease. Other relevant factors are the number of sexual partners, sexually transmitted diseases and prostitution
      D **True**
      E **True**

Brocklehurst, p. 665

9.28 **The following is/are normal age-related changes in the kidney**
- A decrease in kidney weight
- B decrease in glomeruli numbers
- C enlargement of residual nephrons
- D atrophy of afferent glomerular arterioles
- E tubular diverticulae

9.29 **The following is/are characteristic of distal *renal tubular acidosis***
- A urinary sodium greater than 20 mmol/l
- B serum hyperchloraemia
- C normal anion gap metabolic alkalosis
- D urinary sodium greater than 20 mmol/l
- E hypercalcuria

9.30 **Normal age-related *renal* changes include**
- A a marked reduction in renal blood flow
- B invariably a reduction in glomerular function
- C increased sodium retention
- D decreased concentrating ability
- E rising serum creatinine levels

(Answers overleaf)

9.28 A **True**   there is a considerable loss of nephrons with increasing age. This loss of nephrons is reflected in a decrease in kidney weight and loss of parenchymal mass. The average weight of both kidneys at 60 years is 250 g and at 80 years 190 g

    B **True**

    C **True**   as a compensation for the loss and shrinking of the nephrons there is enlargement of the residual nephrons.

    D **True**   the progressive nature of the ageing process is very obvious in the arterial tree. The changes start in the small arteries and arterioles and progress in a centripedal pattern. The renal afferent arteries are the first to undergo changes

    E **True**   the number of diverticulae on the distal convoluted tubule increase with age and may play a part in the production of *pyelonephritis* and in causing recurrence of *renal* infections

Platt, pp 203–206

9.29 A **True**   indicating tubular sodium loss

    B **True**   a hyperchloraemic normal anion gap (Na − (Cl + HCO3) = 10–12 meq) metabolic acidosis suggests either *renal tubular acidosis* or gastrointestinal alkali loss

    C **False**

    D **False**   greater than 20 mmol/l

    E **True**   *hypercalcuria* is consistently present

Cecil, pp 562–563, 574–575

9.30 A **True**   partly dependent or reduced *cardiac output* and partly on the reduction of the cardiovascular bed

    B **False**   even though there is, on average, a decrement in clearance decade by decade even in early adult life, longitudinal studies shows that there are some individuals who show a remarkable maintenance of their renal function. Some show improvement in renal function with age

    C **False**   there is an age related salt losing tendency which can lead to depletion of the extracellular fluid volume when salt intake is reduced

    D **True**   consequently, during limited fluid intake or loss of water aged patients develop volume depletion

    E **False**   because *creatinine* varies with body weight serum levels may not be elevated when renal function is impaired in thin elderly subjects unless corrected appropriately for body weight

Hodkinson, pp 49–50
Platt, pp 205–205

9.31   An uninhibited *bladder*

- A   is common in Parkinson's syndrome
- B   may be diagnosed from a history alone
- C   may be controlled by antispasmodics
- D   always requires catheterisation
- E   is helped by oestrogen therapy

9.32   In *pre-renal azotemia*

- A   urinary sodium concentration is greater than 40 mmol/l
- B   urine osmolality is frequently greater than 500 mosm/kg
- C   the percentage of filtered load of sodium excreted in the urine (Fe_{Na}) is less than 1 per cent.
- D   the urine to plasma urea ratio is less than 3
- E   the urine to plasma creatinine ratio is less than 20

(Answers overleaf)

9.31 A **True**   it is common in *Parkinson's disease*, old age, senile dementia and after cerebrovascular lesions
      B **False**   history alone is generally not sufficient to detect the cause of incontinence and in most cases urodynamic studies are necessary
      C **True**   it may be controlled by antispasmodics, regular voiding by the clock (*bladder drill*), marsupial pads or bladder stretching under anaesthesia
      D **False**   *catheterisation* is only indicated as a 'last resort' in the management of urinary incontinence
      E **True**   oestrogens may help in older women

                                      Jameson, British Medical Journal, 1983

9.32 A **False**   urinary sodium is less than 20 in pre-renal azotemia and greater than 40 in acute tubular necrosis
      B **True**   *urine osmolalities* of less than 350 mosmol/kg and greater than 500 mosmol/kg characterise acute tubular necrosis and pre-renal azotemia respectively
      C **True**   whereas patients with *acute tubular necrosis* frequently have a Fe_{Na} greater than 2 per cent

$$Fe_{Na} \frac{(U/P)\ Na}{(U/P)\ Cr} \times 100$$

      D **False**   a U/P urea ratio of less than 3 is virtually never found in *prerenal azotemia*, whereas values greater than 8 are uncommon in *acute tubular necrosis*
      E **False**   values between 20 and 40 are associated with considerable overlap but values below and above this range differentiate acute tubular necrosis from prerenal azotemia respectively

                                                      Cecil, pp 498–499

9.33   Appropriate treatment of *acute renal failure* includes

A   corticosteroids
B   restriction of salt and water
C   restriction of potassium intake
D   continuous high dose diuretic therapy
E   restriction of protein intake

9.34   Asymptomatic *bacteruria* in the elderly is

A   usually asymptomatic
B   most commonly caused by *Enterobacter coliform*
C   always in need of treatment
D   commoner in females
E   due to proteus infection in 6 per cent of cases

(Answers overleaf)

9.33 A **False**
      B **True**
      C **True**
      D **False**   there is no convincing evidence that continuous high
                      dose *diuretic therapy* favourably alters the course of
                      acute renal failure
      E **True**

                                                    Cecil, pp 499–500

9.34 A **True**
      B **True**   and like many other pathogens producing urinary
                     tract infection, it is mostly derived from the patients
                     own faecal flora. The most common pathway is
                     through the perineum to the periurethral area.
      C **False**   as a general rule, asymptomatic *bacteruria* in the
                     elderly should not be treated. Exceptions to this are
                     the presence of underlying renal disease and proteus
                     infections
      D **True**   in women the enterobacteriaceae which colonise the
                     vagina are frequently identical to those isolated from
                     the urine in patients with recurrent urinary tract
                     infections
      E **True**

                                                    Platt, pp 206–209

10. Rheumatology

10.1 Generalised stiffness is associated with

- A polymyalgia rheumatica
- B haemochromatosis
- C cervical spondylosis and myelopathy
- D Parkinsonism
- E hypothyroidism

10.2 Sudek's atrophy is characteristically associated with

- A osteoarthritis
- B trauma
- C hemiplegia
- D myocardial infarction
- E Paget's disease

10.3 Carpal tunnel syndrome is characteristically associated with

- A myxoedema
- B amyloid
- C rheumatoid arthritis
- D lead poisoning
- E Guillain-Barré syndrome

10.4 A serum uric acid of 0.52 mmol/l in a 75-year-old man is most likely to be due to which of the following

- A a high purine diet
- B Lesch-Nyhan syndrome
- C frusemide
- D chronic renal failure
- E primary gout

(Answers overleaf)

10.1 A **True**
      B **True**
      C **True**
      D **True**
      E **True**   particularly in cold weather. In elderly subjects generalised stiffness is also associated with unaccustomed exercise, systemic infection, rheumatoid arthritis, osteoarthritis, dermatomyositis, scleroderma and any cause of generalised oedema

                                                              Burton, p. 179

10.2 A **False**   it is also characteristically associated with epilepsy,
      B **True**   cervical spinal lesions, brain tumour, pulmonary
      C **True**   lesions, herpes zoster, vasculitis
      D **True**
      E **False**

                                               Cecil, pp 1366, 1885, 1947
                                                              Burton, p. 179

10.3 A **True**
      B **True**
      C **True**
      D **False**
      E **False**

                                                            Cecil, p. 2155
                                                             Burton, p. 180

10.4 A **False**   a high purine diet does cause hyperuricaemia but rarely in this age group
      B **False**   this is an inherited disorder characterised by choreoathetosis, spasticity, mental retardation, self mutilation, excessive production of uric acid, renal stones and renal failure. Death usually occurs in the second of third decade from infection or renal failure
      C **True**
      D **True**
      E **True**
Other causes in this age group are high turnover disease states such as myeloproliferative disease and lymphoma, chronic haemolysis, psoriasis, hyperparathyroidism, salicylates, uricosuric agents, alcohol and hyperlipidaemia

                                                            Cecil, p. 1108

10.5   Paget's disease

A   occurs in 2 per cent of the population over 75 years
B   is characterised by osteoblastic and osteolytic bone activity
C   may be complicated by sensorineural hearing loss
D   is associated with increased blood flow through the external carotid artery
E   is an incidental finding in 80 per cent of cases

10.6   Characteristic features of polymyositis are

A   proximal muscle wasting
B   dysphagia
C   raised plasma creatinine
D   abnormal muscle biopsy
E   early loss of tendon reflexes

10.7   In polymyositis

A   serum compliment levels are elevated
B   the ESR is rarely within the normal range
C   muscle biopsy is normal in over 50 per cent of cases
D   CPK levels are normal in up to 30 per cent of cases
E   high dose steroid therapy is indicated initially

(Answers overleaf)

10.5 A **False**   occurs in 3 per cent of the population under the age of
                     40 and 10 per cent over the age of 70
      B **True**
      C **True**   involvement of the skull results in headaches,
                     intermittent tinnitus, vertigo and hearing loss —
                     usually of the sensorineural type
      D **True**   in patients with severe skull involvement the
                     increased blood flow through the external carotid
                     artery and its branches may contribute to vascular and
                     migraine headaches, as well as pagetic steal
                     syndrome, with symptoms analogous to the
                     subclavian steal syndrome
      E **False**   it is an incidental finding in approximately 20 per cent
                     of cases

                                                          Cecil, p. 1346

10.6 A **True**   with associated pain and tenderness
      B **True**   dysphagia occurs in one third of cases secondary to
                     anterior neck muscle involvement
      C **True**   the plasma creatinine is usually raised, but may be
                     normal in up to 30 per cent of cases
      D **True**   there is evidence of muscle necrosis, phagocytosis
                     and atrophy
      E **False**   loss of tendon reflexes occurs late in the disease

                                              Brocklehurst, pp 828–829
                                             Isenburg, Hospital Update, 1982

10.7 A **False**   serum compliment levels are normal. Serum
                     compliment and antimuscle antibodies have not to
                     date been shown to be toxic
      B **False**   the ESR is normal in 45 per cent
      C **False**   it is normal in up to 15 per cent
      D **True**
      E **False**   recent trials have indicated that 10 mg prednisolone
                     from the start of treatment has the same effect as very
                     high doses (60–100 mg) initially

                                              Brocklehurst, pp 828–829
                                             Isenburg, Hospital Update, 1982

10.8 **Polymyalgia rheumatica is characterised by the following**
- A   peripheral muscle weakness
- B   muscle tenderness
- C   normal ESR
- D   positive rheumatoid factor
- E   joint inflammation

10.9 **The following is/are true of adhesive capsulitis frozen shoulder**
- A   the majority of cases remit spontaneously within 1 month
- B   paracetamol is the best treatment
- C   radiography of the shoulder joint is usually normal
- D   it may occur spontaneously
- E   there is always underlying degenerative joint disease

10.10 **Chondrocalcinosis**
- A   is associated with hypoparathyroidism
- B   occurs in less than 10 per cent of the elderly
- C   is diagnosed by the identification of uric acid crystals in joint aspirates
- D   is associated with haemochromatosis
- E   is associated with Wilson's disease

(Answers overleaf)

10.8   A **False** pain and stiffness usually occur in the girdle and
                     proximal limb muscles
       B **True**   the muscles are usually tender but never weak
       C **False** the ESR is often extremely high, often over 100 mm in
                     the first hour
       D **False** tests for rheumatoid factor are negative
       E **False** there are no objective signs of joint inflammation, viz
                     swelling, tenderness and loss of movement, although
                     there may be coincidental osteoarthrosis.

Many of these cases are shown on temporal artery biopsy to have
indisputable evidence of cranial arteritis. There is no evidence of a
muscle abnormality, and EMG, plasma levels of muscle enzymes and
muscle biopsy are uniformly normal.

Brocklehurst, pp 829–830

10.9   A **False** the majority of cases remit spontaneously within 6 to
                     24 months
       B **False** intra-articular steroids and/or physiotherapy are
                     recommended to relieve pain and stiffness, and both
                     are significantly more effective than the
                     administration of paracetamol alone
       C **True**
       D **True**   it may occur spontaneously or in relation to a variety
                     of predisposing conditions such as trauma, or any
                     painful condition of the upper quadrant of the body
                     which results in a period of immobility of the upper
                     limb. It is commonly seen in old people after
                     myocardial infarction, hemiplegia or pneumonia
       E **False**

Brocklehurst, pp 811–812

10.10 A **False** associated with hyperparathyroidism, Wilson's
                     disease and haemochromatosis
       B **False** *chondrocalcinosis* is present in at least 25 per cent of
                     old people
       C **True**   it is characterised by the presence of calcium-
                     containing salts in cartilaginous structures of joints.
                     These salts include calcium pyrophosphate, calcium
                     hydroxyapatite and calcium orthophosphate
       D **False** idiopathic chondrocalcinosis increases in frequency
                     rapidly with increasing age and is rare below the age
                     of 65. Over the age of 80 years, 25 per cent of surveyed
                     patients have radiological evidence of this condition.
                     The influence of age comes into other aspects of
                     chondrocalcinosis — only older patients with
                     haemochromatosis develop chondrocalcinosis
       E **True**

Brocklehurst, pp 809–810

10.11   The following are associated with vasculitis
    A   osteoarthritis
    B   polyarteritis nodosum
    C   erythema nodosum
    D   cranial arteritis
    E   tuberculosis

10.12   The anaemia of rheumatoid arthritis may be due to
    A   defective iron utilisation
    B   folate deficiency
    C   haemolysis
    D   pernicious anaemia
    E   thalassaemia

10.13   Adhesive capsulitis (frozen shoulder)
    A   is rarely seen in old age
    B   occurs spontaneously
    C   is rarely associated with pain
    D   is characterised by inability to actively elevate the arm
         above the head
    E   remits spontaneously within 12 months

10.14   Acute gouty arthritis
    A   is precipitated by commencing steroid therapy
    B   occurs on the fourth post operative day
    C   responds dramatically to allopurinol
    D   most frequently occurs in the ankle joint
    E   is resistant to colchicine therapy

(Answers overleaf)

10.11 A **False**
    B **True**
    C **True** also *erythema multiformi*, erythema induratum, nodular vasculitis, and some drug rashes
    D **True**
    E **True** associated with an endarteritis obliterans, together with *syphilis*, Buerger's disease and any chronic ulceration, i.e. *peptic ulcer* and *ulcerative colitis*

Burton, p. 178

10.12 A **True** as in *anaemia* of chronic disorders
    B **True**
    C **True** especially in *Felty's syndrome*
    D **True** there is an increased incidence of pernicious anaemia associated with rheumatoid arthritis
    E **False**
It may also be due to iron deficiency, haemodilution, and marrow hypoplasia.

Cecil, p. 843

10.13 A **False** is frequently seen in old age
    B **True** it may occur spontaneously or in relation to a variety of predisposing conditions such as *myocardial infarction*, trauma, *hemiplegia* or pneumonia
    C **False** is characterised by a painful *shoulder* joint, with limited passive movement when the scapula is fixed and inability to actively elevate the arm above the head
    D **True**
    E **True** the vast majority remit spontaneously within 6 to 24 months

Brocklehurst, pp 811–812

10.14 A **False** is precipitated by the cessation of steroids, trauma, surgery, alcohol ingestion, dietary overindulgence, starvation or infection
    B **True** attributed to subsidence of the adrenal alarm
    C **False** colchicine, non steroidal anti-inflammatory agents and/or steroids
    D **False** hallux
    E **False**

Cecil, pp 1112–1117

11. Therapeutics

11.1 The following is/are true of *antibiotic* prophylaxis in patients with valvular heart disease

A   penicillin 24 h before dental surgery
B   gentamycin and metronidazole 6 h before and 6 h after bowel surgery
C   amoxycillin 1 h before and 6 h after catheterisation in a patient with bacteruria
D   a cephalosporin in biliary tract surgery
E   penicillin for hip joint replacement

11.2 The following is/are true of *antibiotic* therapy in the elderly

A   cephaloridine is the least nephrotoxic cephalosporin
B   aminoglycosides should be administered orally
C   toxic effects of aminoglycosides are reduced by concurrent administration of frusemide
D   tetracyclines aggravate renal failure
E   doxycycline is completely excreted in the bile

11.3 The following is/are true of *penicillins* in the elderly

A   oral absorption is enhanced
B   half life of ampicillin is prolonged
C   pulmonary oedema may result from therapy
D   treatment may precipitate hyperkalaemia
E   carbenicillin may cause neurotoxicity

(Answers overleaf)

11.1 A **False**   penicillin should be given 1 h before dental *surgery*. Drugs should be administered immediately before and during the operation and for only a short period thereafter
     B **False**   gentamycin and metronidazole 1 h before and 6 h after bowel surgery.
     C **True**   catheterisation or other operative procedures on the genitourinary tract in patients with bacteruria are potentially hazardous
     D **True**   particularly in the elderly and in obstructive disease
     E **False**   a cephalosporin or penicillinase-resistant penicillin are appropriate

                                                             Harrison, p. 917

11.2 A **False**   cephaloridine is not recommended for use in old age because of reduced renal function
     B **False**   aminoglycosides are administered parenterally and therefore careful monitoring of peak (30 min after i.v. dose) and trough (30 min before next dose) levels is necessary
     C **False**   toxic effects of aminoglycosides are enhanced by concurrent administration of potent loop diuretics such as frusemide and ethacrynic acid
     D **True**   and are hepatotoxic
     E **True**

                                                             Brocklehurst, pp 95–96

11.3 A **True**   because of increasing achlorhydria
     B **True**   glomerular filtration rate is lower and tubular capacity reduced in old age therefore the half-life of ampicillin is prolonged
     C **True**   the *penicillins* can contain large amounts of sodium or potassium which may precipitate *pulmonary oedema* or *hyperkalaemia*
     D **True**
     E **True**   this is one of the rarer side-effects of penicillins which is more common in the elderly; others include *neurotoxicity* with ticarcillin or penicillin G, hypokalaemic alkalosis with penicillin G, and interference with coagulation by carbenicillin

                                                             Brocklehurst, p. 95

11.4 *Tardive dyskinesia*
  A is rarely associated with facial movement
  B complicates long-term administration of dopamine
     antagonists
  C is commonly seen in schizophrenia
  D may persist for months after drug withdrawal
  E is precipitated by L-dopa therapy in normal individuals

11.5 **The following is/are true of** *ototoxicity*
  A neomycin is vestibulotoxic
  B tobramycin is cochleotoxic
  C gentamycin is vestibulotoxic
  D ethacrynic acid is vestibulotoxic
  E practolol may cause otitis media

(Answers overleaf)

11.4 A **False**   repetitive stereotypical movements frequently involve the face, tongue, and extremities
      B **False**   it is a complication of administration of *dopamine* antagonists and probably results from hypersensitivity of either presynaptic or postsynaptic dopamine receptors in the striatum resulting from prolonged treatment with antagonists
      C **True**
      D **True**   it may persist for months or years after drug withdrawal
      E **False**   excessive leva-dopa therapy in *Parkinson's* disease may induce a wide variety of abnormal movements that seem to be dose related. It does not have this effect on normal individuals. Presumably, certain striatal neurons, other than the ones causing the Parkinson's syndrome have been rendered hypersensitive

                                                                Harrison, p. 94

11.5 A **False**
      B **True**
      C **True**   it is also *cochleotoxic*
      D **False**   cochleotoxic — the diuretic ethacrynic acid causes loss of outer hair cells in the cochlea with an irreversible hearing loss
      E **True**   practolol may cause a serious otitis media

                                                             Brocklehurst, p. 95

References

Bahemuka M, Hodkinson HM (1975)
Screening for hypothyroidism in elderly inpatients.
British Medical Journal 2: 601–603

Bird AC (1983) Laser photocoagulation of senile macular degeneration.
British Medical Journal 286: 1001

Brocklehurst JC (1984)
Textbook of Geriatric Medicine. 3rd edn, Churchill Livingstone,
Edinburgh

Burton JL (1983)
Aids to postgraduate Medicine. 4th edn, Churchill Livingstone,
Edinburgh

Caird CI (1982)
Neurology of Old Age. 1st edn, Wright PC, London

Campbell AJ, Reinken J, Allan BC, Martinez GS (1981)
Falls in old age: a study of frequency and related clinical features.
Age and Ageing 10: 264–270

Cecil (1982)
Textbook of Medicine, (ed Wyngaarden JB, Smith LH) 16th edn, WB
Saunders Company, Philadelphia

de Gruchy GC (1978)
Clinical Haematology in Medical Practice
(ed Penington D, Rush B, Castaldi P)
4th edn, Blackwell Scientific Publications, Oxford

Editorial (1977)
Communicating hydrocephalus.

Faizallah R, Green HT, Krasner N, Walker RJ (1982)
Outbreak of chicken pox from a patient with immunosuppressed
herpes zoster in hospital.
British Medical Journal 285: 1022–1023
Lancet 2: 1011–1012

Flear CTG, Gill GV, Burn J (1981)
Hyponatraemia: mechanisms and management.
Lancet 2: 26–31

George CF (1983)
Digitalis intoxication.

Godfrey JW, Roberts MA, Caird FI (1982)
Epileptic seizures in the elderly: 11 Diagnostic problems 11: 29–34
British Medical Journal 286: 1533–1534

Godfrey JW, Roberts MA, Caird FI (1982) Epileptic seizures in the
    elderly. Diagnostic Problems 11: 29–34
Gosling HR, Pellegrini VD (1982)
    Fat embolism syndrome: a review of the pathophysiology and
    physiological basis of treatment.
    Clinical Orthopaedics 165: 68–82
Harrison Petersdorf RG, Adams RD, Brau dwald E, Isselbacher KJ,
    Martin JB, Wilson J. ed. (1983) Principles of Internal Medicine 10th
    edn, McGraw-Hill Book Company, New York
Hodkinson H17 (1984) Clinical Biochemistry in the Elderly. Churchill
    Livingstone, Edinburgh
Impallomeni M, Kenny RA, Flynn MD, Kraenzlin M, Pallis C (1984)
    The elderly and their ankle jerks Lancet 1: 670–672
Isenburg D, Cambridge G (1982) Polymyositis. Hospital Update
    8: 639–646
Jameson RM (1983).
    Incontinence in women with neuropathic bladder.
    British Medical Journal 287: 627–628
Kafetz K, Cox M (1982)
    Alcohol excess and the senile squalor syndrome.
    Journal of the American Geriatrics Society 30: 706
Kenny RA (1982)
    Epilepsy — its diagnosis and management.
    Geriatric Medicine 12: 61–62
Kenny RA (1984)
    The significance of a long QT interval.
    Postgraduate Medical Journal (in press)
Kenny RA, Timmers J, Kafetz K, Cox M, Impallomeni M (1984a)
    Impaired nitrazepam metabolism in hypothyroidism. Age and
    Ageing 60: 57–58
Kenny RA, Cox M, Caspi D, Hodkinson HM, Pepys MB (1984b)
    The acute phase protein response to infection in elderly patients. Age
    and Ageing 13: 89–94
Kenny RA, Stephens S, Hodkinson HM (1984c) Hatchinski Ischaemic
    Score in demented elderly patients. Journal Clinical Experimental
    Gerontology 63–74
Kenny RA, Hodkinson HM, Prendiville A, Hayes M, Flynn MD (1984c)
    Abnormalities of Liver Function and the predictive value of lives
    function tests in infection and outcome of acutely ill elderly patients.
    Age and Ageing 13: 224–229
Kenny RA, Saunders A, Coll A, Harrington M, Caspi D, Hodkinson HM,
Pepys M (1985)
    A comparison of the erythrocyte sedimentation rate and C reactive
    protein in elderly patients. Age and Ageing (in press)
Mellström D, Rundgren Å, Svanberg A (1981)
    Previous alcohol consumption and its consequences for ageing,
    morbidity and mortality in men aged 70–75. Age and Ageing 10:
    277–286

McEvoy A, Dutton J, James OFW (1983)
    Bacterial contamination of the small intestine is an important cause
    of occult malabsorption in the elderly.
    British Medical Journal 287: 789–793
Oakley CM (1983)
    After Infarct. British Medical Journal 287: 625
Pallis C (1983)
    ABC of Brain stem death.
    British Medical Journal 286: 39, 123
Perry RH, Blessed G, Perry EK, Tomlinson BE (1980)
    Histochemical observations in cholinesterase activities in the brains
    of elderly and demented (alzheimer-type) patients. Age and Ageing
    9: 9–16
Platt D (1983)
    Geriatrics 2. Springer Verlag, Berlin
Price NC (1983)
    Importance of asking about glaucoma.
    British Medical Journal 286: 349
Price (1978)
    The practice of medicine (ed Sir R Bodley Scott), 12th edn, Oxford
    University Press, Oxford
Roberts MA, Godfrey JW, Caird FI (1982)
    Epileptic seizures in the elderly: 1 aetiology and type of seizure. Age
    and Ageing 11: 24–28
Weksler BB, Lewin M (1983)
    Anticoagulation in cerebral ischaemia.
    Stroke 14: 658–663